Leadership Laboratory
for Nurse Leaders

Leadership Laboratory for Nurse Leaders

Barbara Mackoff, Ed.D.

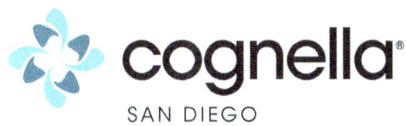

cognella®
SAN DIEGO

Bassim Hamadeh, CEO and Publisher
Amanda Martin, Publisher
Amy Smith, Senior Project Editor
Rachel Kahn, Production Editor
Jess Estrella, Senior Graphic Designer
Kylie Bartolome, Licensing Associate
Ursina Kilburn, Interior Designer
Stephanie Adams, Senior Marketing Program Manager
Natalie Piccotti, Director of Marketing
Kassie Graves, Senior Vice President, Editorial
Jamie Giganti, Director of Academic Publishing

Cover image copyright © 2014 iStockphoto LP/IPGGutenbergUKLtd.
Interior design images:
Source: Adapted from https://uxwing.com/magnifier-glass-icon/.
Source: Adapted from https://uxwing.com/chemistry-flask-icon/.
Source: Adapted from https://uxwing.com/scuba-diving-icon/.
Source: Adapted from https://uxwing.com/bulb-light-icon/.
Source: Adapted from https://uxwing.com/question-mark-round-line-icon/.

Chapters 1-6 of this book grew from the process of writing a number of columns for the Nurse Leader, a publication of American Organization of Nursing Leaders (AONL). Copyright © by American Organization for Nursing Leadership (AONL). Used with permission.

Printed in the United States of America.

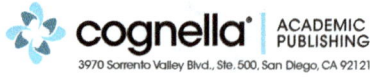
cognella® ACADEMIC PUBLISHING
3970 Sorrento Valley Blvd., Ste. 500, San Diego, CA 92121

For Sam and Selma Mackoff

And always, for Hannah and Jeremy

Knowing is not enough; we must apply.

Willing is not enough; we must do.

Johann Von Goethe

Brief Contents

Detailed Contents

Foreword

Leadership is a journey, not an event. It is a lifelong process of learning, adapting, and transforming. Newer concepts generated from complexity science (quantum leadership) are now informing us about how leadership works at the intersection of complex adaptive human systems, and how it needs to be expressed at every place in the human experience. This means that, at some time or other, everyone in the human community will need to demonstrate some capacity for leadership. Fortunately for us all, leadership is always a learned skill.

Leadership is not complex. Instead, the circumstances within which leadership must be expressed are often complex. The talent of a great leader lies in the ability to know what that context is, and to determine the appropriate response to it. In the sixth century, Lao Tsu proclaimed, "A leader is best when people barely know he exists, when his work is done, his aim fulfilled, they will say: we did it ourselves." He was one of the earliest social scholars to understand the implications of complexity in societies and the simplicity of the principles of leadership in navigating the shoals of relationships and shared experiences.

Leadership is lived in the moment, but is practiced over a lifetime. Embedded in this understanding is the realization that each of us are owners of our lives, and that the good leader neither impedes nor robs anyone of this ownership. In fact, leaders enable ownership and serve as a catalyst for its full expression. It is this act of enabling others' full expression of their talents, skills, learnings, experiences, and lives, and the convergence of that energy in a community of engagement, that truly advances the human condition. This understanding underscores Lao Tsu's insight about leadership and the empowerment of others' expression of it, such that its expression remains unnoticed in its subtlety. We are aware of it instead in its impact, outcome, and inside the transformational moment ("we did it ourselves"). Good leadership in this context is a recognition, an awareness that comes to us on arrival. It is the demonstration of positive impact that is the evidence of effective leadership—and it often has no words. It is instead an appreciation of having arrived in a better place where we are enhanced, made better, growing and becoming.

Warren Bennis and others suggest that "great leaders don't set out to be a leader ... they set out to make a difference." Leadership is not a position one occupies; it is instead an expression, a process, a practice. One knows leaders in what they do, in how that reveals who they are and who you are. These persons are filled with a passion in their lives in a way that represents their engagement of purpose. The good leader lives "in the question," always searching, pushing boundaries and drilling down to the "why" in an effort to reveal meaning and purpose. The leader knows that value in life is discovered, not defined, and that there is a good fit between meaning and action if that value is to ever be advanced and sustained. Leadership behavior and practice is not itself leadership; instead it is the demonstration of leadership and the evidence of its presence. Leadership practices proceed from the knowledge, insight, and character of the leader. These behaviors are not ends but are instead means. Evidence of their success is found in the veracity and sustainability of action and outcome. What makes leadership great is the authenticity and transparency of the leader in all they are and do on the leadership journey.

It is this understanding of leadership as a journey that best underpins the insights and practices detailed in this book. Barbara has broken through the myths and complexity historically attached to leadership, and identified the practices that most demonstrate its successful exercise. She understands the inner work of reflection, translation, application, and evaluation, and indeed makes them the work of leader development. Grounding leadership practices in everyday lived experience and clinical practice scenarios, Barbara makes them real, habitual, and a fundamental part of acting and relating every day. The author's sustaining use of the discipline of learning, reflection, experiment, and reflection again makes practical the flow of dynamics on the leadership learning trajectory. This methodology helps focus the mind and make the process of application intentional in a way that assures a growing level of competence and an awareness of progress. In addition, a discipline is established that makes leadership moments conscious, transparent, and subject to adjustment and recalibration, serving as a vehicle for continuous learning. This mindfulness becomes a part of the practice of leadership and keeps open the mind and heart to the unending possibilities bundled in advancing common purpose and collective relationships.

The elements and exercises of leadership in this book reflect a lifetime of accrued and collected wisdom gained from real-life experiences and exemplary leadership teaching and learning. Practices are connected to the shared insights of many contemporary leadership scholars and practitioners, and are sewn into the exemplars and experiments of leadership expression. Each chapter becomes a real-time tool chest of relevant and tested approaches to effective leadership, interaction, and communion in a format that is timeless in its approach. Using these resources, the learning leader can return to elements in each chapter repeatedly and gain new insights and strategies for addressing the ever-changing landscape of human effort, on an unending path of advancement and growth.

With this resource, the never-ending and ever-exciting challenges of leading and leadership become doable, practical, possible. In addition, the leader develops and demonstrates her or his own wisdom and becomes a beacon for others in their own leadership journey, ever building and enhancing our human community. It is to this end that this book is especially relevant, and is most recommended to all of us as we live through our moments of leadership, wherever and whenever they are needed in our own life's journey. Ultimately, at some point along our way, we will all be leaders. This book can help you succeed at it.

Tim Porter-O'Grady
Senior Partner, TPOG Associates, LLC
Clinical Professor, Emory University School of Nursing

Acknowledgments

For me, writing acknowledgments is a meaningful closing ceremony—the opportunity to celebrate and appreciate both the book's completion and the circle of support that has surrounded me.

I want to honor the storytellers on these pages, the nurse leaders around the world who shared vivid experiences of their challenges, triumphs, and strategies in learning to lead. The stories sing with vulnerability and authority; they translate theory into practice.

I treasure the wise kindness of Tim Porter O-Grady. First, for his matchmaking introduction to my editor, Amanda Martin at Cognella, and then for writing a most thoughtful and gracious foreword.

Amanda, thank you for the way you immediately understood my direction and diction in the book and for being a steadfast kindred spirit. Special thanks to my Cognella team: project editor Amy Smith for her good humored guidance, clarity, and patience; graphic designer Jess Estrella for a striking and inviting cover; production editors Rachel Kahn and Alia Bales for expertly guiding me through the weeds of revisions; copyeditor Trista Smith for her close reading of the manuscript; and Stephanie Adams for her shiny ideas for bringing this book to market.

I also want to recognize and thank the nurse leaders who were early adopters of leadership laboratories in their organizations. Kim Glassman at NYU Langone Medical Center, Rosanne Raso and Irene Macyk at Lenox Hill Hospital, Cole Edmondson at Dallas Presbyterian Hospital, and Sidsel Rasborg Wied at Gentofte Hospital in Denmark.

I am ever grateful to my colleagues at the American Organization of Nursing Leaders (AONL): Pamela Thomson for her kaleidoscopic thinking and generativity; Teresa Thrall, who skillfully edited my leadership laboratory columns in *Nurse Leader*; Beverly Hancock, my partner in the excitement of creating the first online leadership laboratory for AONL; and Crystal Lawson, my valued counterpart in conducting the ongoing leadership labs.

It was a pleasure to explore the Finnish art of Sisu with the brilliant and ever gracious Emilia Elisabet Lahti. Thank you Lisa Peters for sharing your team of story tellers.

And special thanks to AONL CEO Robyn Begley and COO Matt Fenwick, as well as Danielle Ward and Beverly Hancock for working with me to create a means to channel all of my proceeds from this book to a new scholarship fund for the AONL Nurse Fellowship Program.

I have been buoyed by the encouragement of Jane Adams, Kate Marrone, and Ray Karesky. I cherish the elevating support and insights of my home team—Jeremy, Hannah, and Ezra—my first readers and most beloved cheerleaders.

Introduction

The book you hold in your hands was designed to place you at the busy intersection between evidence-based literature and your lived experiences. In each chapter, you will be prompted to view your experiences of learning to lead through the lens of new and established ideas in the literature of nursing, psychology, education, sociology, and anthropology. You will use your unique experiences to bring these literatures to life by responding to a series of reflective exercises.

And there is more. Each chapter encourages you to experiment with new strategies drawn from expert research. Every topic also includes more than a dozen examples of peer successes and challenges—suggesting strategic best practices, emotional insights, and exemplary models for meeting the demands of being in charge.

A Little History

The seeds of a leadership laboratory were planted more than decade ago with a meeting of minds and intentions in my collaboration with Kimberly Glassman, chief nursing officer (CNO) at New York University Langone Medical Center.[1] Kim wanted to express her support for a group of 40 nurse managers and to invest in their development in leadership roles. "Standard training and seminars don't have much effect," she told me. Could we create a fresh format for leadership development—design a process distinct from a standard-issue seminar experience?

Kim's question was catnip for me. My colleague, Pamela Triolo, and I had just completed a nationwide interview- and narrative-based study of engaged exemplary nurse managers, funded by The Robert Wood Johnson Foundation.[2] Having submitted the requisite research papers, I was now eager to imagine a learning environment that centered on the discussion of peer stories and leadership lessons.

We mapped out a pilot program. Research director Wendy Budin joined the team to track our outcomes. We began with a unique goal: to capture participant nurse managers' lived experiences and best practices in learning to lead—and use them to shape a peer-driven educational process.

The initial leadership laboratories (time management in light of mission, change and resilient thinking, self-regulation, conflict and communication) were organized around activities that maximized self-reflection, peer-to-peer consultation, and best practice narratives.

Case example homework narratives (personal challenge descriptions) were assigned for each meeting and would be the focus of discussion in the session. For each topic, I would present theory and strategy from various literatures. The group would then engage with these ideas by using reflection, storytelling, mutual advising, suggestions of practice strategies, and problem brainstorming.

Our extensive evaluation of the project tracked significant and sustained learning, and the application of ideas and strategies introduced in the laboratories. A year later, when asked to rank the most important elements of the laboratory process, participants gave high marks to learning best practices from peers, self-knowledge, and sharing about day-to-day experiences.

Over time, the dynamics of the laboratory process have been developed and polished in a variety of settings. Examples include an 18-month leadership development program at Lenox Hill Hospital in New York with CNOs Rosanne Raso and Irene Macyk and the expansion of leadership laboratories classrooms to a self-sustaining learning community with CNO Cole Edmondson at Texas Health Presbyterian in Dallas.[3]

As a Fulbright specialist, I had the opportunity to design and facilitate leadership laboratories with nurse managers and directors at Gentofte Hospital in Hellerup, Denmark, and Helsinki University Hospital in Finland.[4] I am currently working to develop laboratories for directors and managers at Zurich University Hospital in Switzerland.

For the last 8 years (with the initial enthusiasm of American Organization of Nursing Leadership Chief Executive Officer Emeritus Pam Thompson), Senior Program Manager Beverly Hancock and Education Director Crystal Lawson have been my essential partners in crafting an online AONL national leadership laboratory.

All of this work was anchored by two theories of practice, which support each chapter in translating the leadership laboratory experience into this workbook format.

Two Theoretical Anchors

Reflective Practice: The Experience of Surprise

The current consensus that reflection jumpstarts learning in nursing practice was first glimpsed in the journals of Florence Nightingale[5, 6]—who would have been a prolific blogger—and grounded in the work of educator John Dewey.[7]

The literature of reflective practice gathered steam in the late 1970s in the widely read work of Carper[8] (personal, aesthetic, and ethical ways of knowing), followed by Schön[9] ("reflection on-action and in action"), and Benner[10] ("knowing how" and "knowing that").

The key assumption and aspiration of these influential writings was that reflection creates a kind of infrastructure—a sturdy bridge between knowledge and experience. In this view, change will result as a by-product of the search for insight.[11] In the decades that followed, nurse educators and researchers expanded these ideas to fashion new understandings and applications of reflective practice.

The acts involved in reflection were identified and name-checked. Among them were describing experience, casting back, analyzing, exploring knowledge bases, questioning assumptions and values, mining underlying emotions, and adaptive change planning. A variety of reflective tools, including cue questions, poetry, journaling, painting, and drawing, were suggested.[12, 13, 14, 15, 16, 17, 18, 19, 20]

More recently, reflection has been elaborated on as an educational strategy in nursing leadership education.[21, 22] Practitioners and researchers have drawn upon reflective practice as the source of juicy lessons for leaders' self-development and enhanced emotional competence, including the understanding of core values and assumptions.[23]

In these studies, the explorations of reflection are seen to mirror elements of leadership capacity, including self-awareness, self-appraisal, analysis, and the generation of new perspectives.

Coward's descriptions of reflection as a fruitful, if not always comfortable, exploration captures the spirit of this book. She writes, "The thinking and unpacking element of reflection ideally reveals a wealth of discomfort and further questioning."[24] Such new understandings and appreciations are something Schön called "the experience of surprise."[25]

That said, constructive caveats about reflective practice research have raised crucial questions. Does insight (alone) lead to behavior change? Does inner work change outer behavior? Are we creating reflection fatigue among students and nurse leaders? Could reflective prompts restrict critical thinking?[26, 27]

Mindful of these queries, we will be inspired by Thompson and Pascal's call to expand Schön's contrast of reflection-on-action and in-action. They underline the importance of foresight and planning—"reflection **for** action."[28]

Since leaders do not develop by reflection alone, this kind of action orientation is central to your work on these pages. In each chapter, reflective prompts alternate with behavioral suggestions and peer best practices. Your invitations to reflect will also include considerations of both challenges and successes.

In other words, we will heed Nurse Nightingale's pithy advice: "Deed not creed." And yet, there are tales to be told. Because the major tool of reflection is storytelling, born of lived experience.

When Phenomenology Meets Andragogy: Lived Experiences and Sticky Stories

Our seven leadership laboratories offer a process where the philosophy of phenomenology (exploring lived experience)[29] swipes right for the methods of andragogy (designing adult education).[30] Translation: to engage adult nurse leaders—who bring a great volume of experience to the table—learning must be grounded in relevance to real-life events, tasks, and relationships.

In each chapter, the use of reflective storytelling prompts will ask you to describe and explore the meaning of your experiences. The richness of reflective practice narratives in leadership education has been convincingly demonstrated in research that maps situational analysis of storied leadership lessons.[31, 32, 33, 34]

Your work here is supported by the understanding that narratives of your day-to-day lives are also accounts of learning that can be leveraged into wisdom. Values, priorities, and codes of conduct can be revealed in your stories. Painful and elevating events can become commitments. Stories of success suggest actions and attitudes to carry forward. Mistakes become research, rather than failures.

In my own adventures as a consulting psychologist and educator for the last 35 years, I have discovered that stories are sticky. We each bring our own history and memories when we listen to the lived experiences of others. Stories beget stories.

In this way, the peer wise practice narratives in each chapter will enable you to be resources to each other. These accounts of learning from nurse leaders around the world are meant to enliven your imagination and memory; to move you to remember the times, places, and people that drove home vital lessons.

As you open a window to view how your colleagues have made sense of their experiences, I want to draw you back to the consequential people and moments in your practice. I intend for you to draw actionable strategies from these stories and also to use the peer narratives as a mirror—to enable you to capture instructive truths about your own experiences as a leader.

How to Use This Book

The subjects of the first six chapter-laboratories (wisdom of experience, motivation, boundary clarity, self-regulation, generativity, and change agility) were chosen as explorations of some crucial elements of emotional mastery for nurse leaders. A final chapter, introducing the Finnish practice of sisu, grew out of my four summers of working with nurse leaders at Helsinki University Hospital.

Each chapter is divided into four sections. The first is a narrative summary of key topic ideas and critical research. It includes invitations and prompts for reflection marked by the symbol 🔍 . It also features experiments, marked with the symbol 🧪 . These are suggestions of new behaviors sourced from expert counsel.

The second section, Peer Wise Ideas, offers stories in the words of leaders, including specific strategies and outlooks. You will be encouraged to explore the resonant lessons in your leadership practice that come to mind as you read these stories.

The third section, Q & Q, is a series of quotes with questions to prompt further reflection about your own experiences that relate to the chapter topic. The fourth section, Deep Dive, lists professional journals, books, videos, and podcasts for further study.

A final thought: By now, you have probably noticed that although the workbook is situated in research traditions, the tone is casual and conversational. This reveals a not-so-secret devotion in my work. I believe that leadership development must be challenging and rigorous, but it need not be tedious. I want you to enjoy—and to be elevated by—your adventures in learning to lead.

Barbara L. Mackoff, EdD
Seattle, Washington
May 10, 2022

Wise Leadership

Learn From Experience

"I came to the ER with an East Coast style of management, in terms of making split-second decisions for critical and clinical reasons. I got tremendous resistance in the beginning [because] I was perceived as abrupt, rash, disrespectful, for things that I was oblivious to. I am very, very patient care oriented; I didn't care if I hurt your feelings if it was going to save a patient. So I had to learn how not to sacrifice that, but get the message across in a different way."

A West Coast nurse manager

◇◇◇◇◇◇◇◇◇◇◇◇◇◇◇◇◇◇

Your colleague from two coasts teaches us that the practice of wisdom—and the proof that you have learned from experience—is a change in behavior. In this chapter, we will explore the two key elements in the practice of wise leadership she has described: how to make sense of your experiences, and then, how to leverage those insights to create the understanding of self and others that drives growth and behavior change.

Polymath playwright Johann Von Goethe summarized this dual assignment when he wrote, "It is not enough to know; we must apply."

Wise leadership is a strategy of inner work that asks you to think again. It is a hybrid of reflective practice that organizes the future with an eye to the recent past. Leaders who learn from their experiences understand that their lessons are not about shame, blame, or claims to fame; they are opportunities to engage in strategic planning.

Let's begin with theologian James Loder's observation that knowing is an event.[1] Initial reflection yields one or more convincing insights. The critical question is whether these insights lead to new commitments. Did your aha! moment become a distant memory? Did you "get it" and forget it? Or does your understanding yield long-term changes and enrich your leadership?

REFLECTION

Describe a time when you faced a major disappointment, an unhappy surprise, or made a significant error in judgment. How did you explain the situation? What was your most convincing insight? Did you (or how could you) carry that learning forward? Did it result in a commitment to think or act differently?

....

....

....

....

....

Next, describe a time when you resolved a problem or accomplished a goal. What were your insights about your success? Did you (or could you) carry that learning into your practice?

....

....

....

....

....

Four Keys to Leveraging Lessons From Your Leadership

Examine four keys to finding meaning, and making sense of your missteps and successes, as well as ideas for applying those lessons in your leadership. As you read, continue to reflect on your experiences and compare your lessons with the ones that follow. Identify your best practices and learning strategies and plan to experiment with some new actions.

Key	Strategies	Your best practices
Key #1 Compose the event.	~Argue with your assumptions. ~Practice the rule of six. ~Don't get lost in the details. ~Use perceptual positioning.	
Key #2 Lead with your questions.	~Pull up the roots. ~Uncover your participation. ~Engage in reflection that leads to action. ~Ask: What? Why? And now what?	
Key #3 Don't fight the feedback.	~Drill down the details. ~Mind the gap between intention and action. ~Discover déjà vu. ~Don't get back on your horse.	
Key #4 Study success as carefully as missteps.	~Adapt a growth mindset. ~Conduct a success audit. ~Discipline your memory.	

Key #1: Compose the Event

Psychologist Robert Kegan suggests that learning from experience begins in the interaction between an event and our reaction to it.[2] We privately compose and frame events, and then we react to them, based on the meaning we have made. These moments of meaning, explains Kegan, can provide crisp insight and calls to action. On the other hand, our compositions contain more sour notes than grace notes when they are drowned out by the noise of previous assumptions, and distorted by memories past of experiences.

This was the case with Eloise D., a nurse leader who sat down with what she called "yet another irresponsible teenage mother." As they talked, this 17-year-old patient described her birth plan, the involvement of the father, and her plan to continue school. Now Eloise understood the situation with a different meaning. "I was so wrong. She was a very mature young woman. I assumed I knew 'her type.' In the future, I won't assume anything and remember that each situation is different."

As Eloise learned, making sense can require an argument with your beliefs and assumptions. Psychologist Gary Klein, whose extensive studies of the nature of insight describe how our core beliefs anchor the way we interpret events.[3] We get trapped—and shut down insights—when we stick to just one story. Insight, explains Klein, is a better story (or, Kegan might add, a better song).

Eloise understood that she had misread her patient by drawing upon assumptions and stories of other irresponsible young moms. As a result, she told a better story—that each person is an individual. Our compositions and storytelling improve when we can explore our distortion by considering alternative points of view.

REFLECTION

Describe an experience with a team member, colleague, or patient where your beliefs and assumptions—drawn from previous experience—affected your judgment or distorted your understanding.

....

....

....

....

....

Next, rethink the experience using two thought experiments.

EXPERIMENT

Educator Paula Underwood Spencer has written about an Iroquois thought practice called The Rule of Six (RO6).[4] It is a strategy to keep biases in check and prevent you from locking into one way of making sense. Here's the drill: For every experience, try to come up with six plausible explanations. One student of management who began using RO6 reported, "It really helped me learn about how my staff might see things differently than I do."

Revise the assumption experience described above by using RO6: Note six possible alternate explanations beyond your original assumptions.

1. ....
   ....

2. ....
   ....

3. ....
   ....

4. ....
   ....

5. ....
   ....

6. ....
   ....

Consider Salvador Dali's painting *Still Life—Fast Moving.*

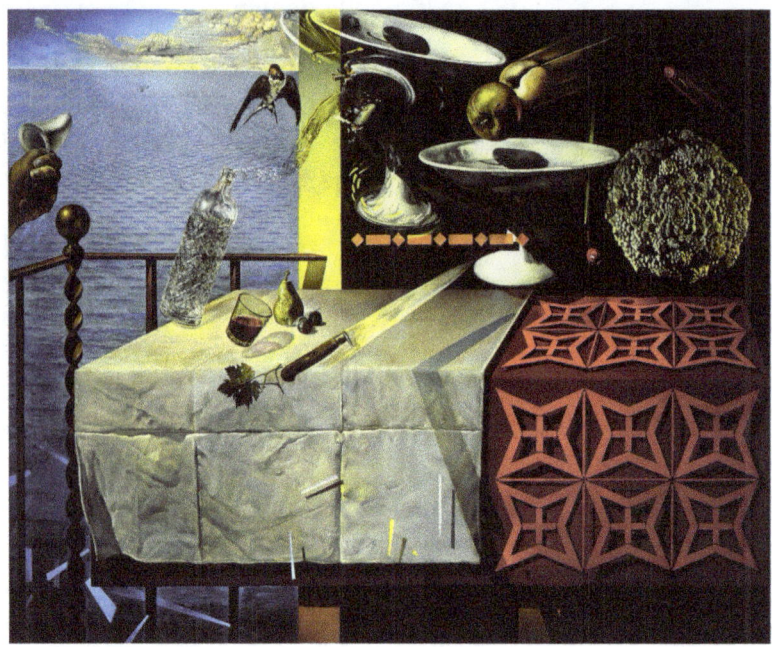

FIGURE 1.1

When you studied the painting, did you focus on specific details (a knife floating above the table) rather than the bigger picture (what is causing the objects to hover above the table)? Similarly, we tend to concentrate on small details ("And then she said, and then I said ...") instead of the larger lessons and questions that could inform or guide us.

....

....

....

....

Return to your previous story of assumptions. What were the details? What were the larger questions and lessons?

....

....

....

....

....

EXPERIMENT

Anthropologist Gregory Bateson and neurolinguistic programmers John Griner and Judith De Lozier pioneered the strategy of perceptual positioning.[5] This requires reconstructing events from three distinct vantage points. The first position is the way you think and feel based on how you view the situation. The second position is a stance of reversibility, of seeing, hearing, and feeling the situation as if you were the other person or people involved. The third position is a fly-on-the-wall view. What would you see, think, or feel if you were an uninvolved person?

....

....

....

....

....

Revisit your experience from these three vantage points:

What do you think and feel based on how you view the situation?

....

....

....

....

....

What would you see, hear, and feel about the situation if you were the other person or people involved?

....

....

....

....

What would you see, think, or feel if you were an uninvolved person—a fly on the wall?

....

....

....

....

....

REFLECTION

Describe what you learned about the event, and about yourself, by using RO6 and perceptual positioning.

....

....

....

....

....

Key #2: Lead With Your Questions

The wisdom of experience is grounded in the art of the questions you ask. Let's review your bicoastal colleague's leadership lesson above by pulling up the root causes of her conflict via the Six Sigma strategy of the five whys.[6]

Her staff saw her abrupt and disrespectful. *Why?* Because she had a different style than they were used to. *Why?* Because in her previous position on the East Coast she had made valuable split-second decisions. *Why?* Because clinical and critical care issues were always at stake. *Why?* Because her goal was to save the patient and not shield the staff members' feelings. *Why?* Because her ethics put the patient first.

Only when she questioned why staff resisted her style was she able to discover that "the communication here was not only that you had to be very careful in how you spoke, what your face looked like, what you did with your hands, how fast you made an answer." As she explained, her wise reflection allowed her "to be able to be comfortable with my own skin, keep my standards, and yet deliver the message with a manner that could be accepted."

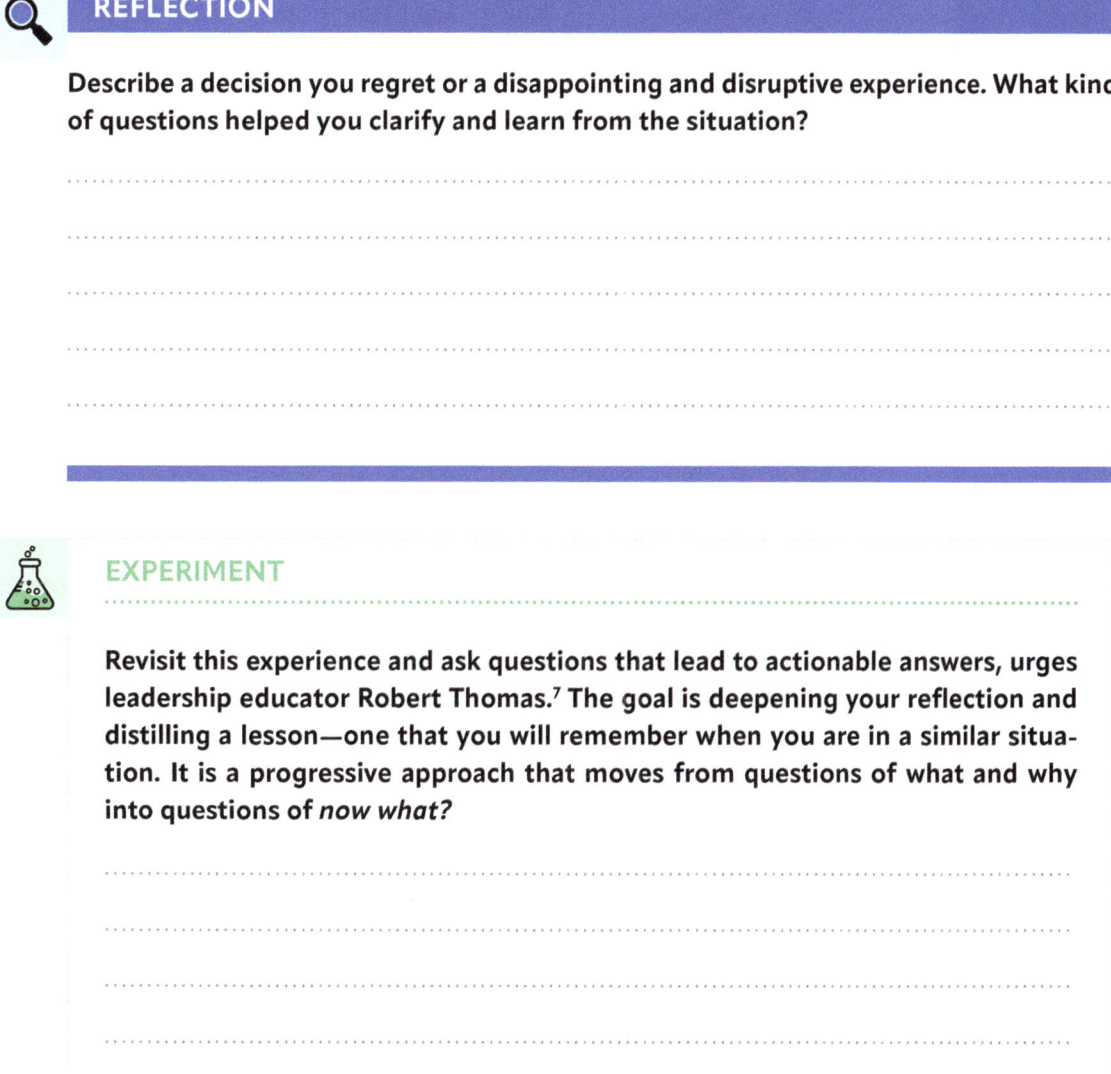

REFLECTION

Describe a decision you regret or a disappointing and disruptive experience. What kind of questions helped you clarify and learn from the situation?

EXPERIMENT

Revisit this experience and ask questions that lead to actionable answers, urges leadership educator Robert Thomas.[7] The goal is deepening your reflection and distilling a lesson—one that you will remember when you are in a similar situation. It is a progressive approach that moves from questions of what and why into questions of *now what?*

Create new meaning by answering these questions about the experience you described.

Why did this happen?

....

....

....

....

....

Why did this happen to me?

....

....

....

....

....

What would I want to teach someone else?

....

....

....

....

....

How could this situation have ended in a different way?

....

....

....

....

....

Is there information I have now that would have been helpful then?

....

....

....

....

....

How can I avoid getting in this situation again?

....

....

....

....

....

What do I want to start doing or stop doing?

....

....

....

....

....

 REFLECTION

Ask questions that point to your participation in creating a problem. Hanne R. explains, "I want to own my part, to have the outcome be more important than me. Part of [this] is a self-check, part of it is being able to learn and to use my peers, or witnesses, to say, 'that is not where I wanted to go, did you see where it got off track, [or] I'm not sure what I said.'"

Add these queries to explore the problematic situation you described:

How did I co-create or participate in this problem situation?

....

....

....

....

....

And, when you succeed, don't forget to ask, how did I contribute to this positive outcome?

....

....

....

....

....

Key #3: Don't Fight the Feedback

Listening to negative feedback—whether it is delivered in a sensitive or scorching manner—creates a tug of war between your desire to be appreciated and your desire to learn. In terms of accepting feedback, nobody did it better than Groucho Marx, who famously responded to a nasty barb by admitting, "I resemble that remark."

Learning from feedback casts you in the dual role of a participant and observer. Only by understanding how others see you can you learn how your behavior affects them. You can discover the difference between what you intend and the impact it has on others.

Fred B. offers a master class in accepting and learning from feedback. He describes his habit of entering the unit each morning preoccupied with an edgy email or an unresolved issue. He admits, "When I arrived at my unit, I never took the time to ask our night shift how their shift went or if there were any issues I needed to help them with. I just began my rant." Then two well-regarded members of his staff came to his office and told Fred that he never asked them anything about their shift. They explained that the day for them ended with an angry unit director on top of an already stressful night.

Fred knew that he resembled their remarks. He thanked them both for the feedback and for being brave enough to tell him that he was falling short as a leader. He translated his lesson into the practice of beginning his day with rounding on the night shift and asking specific questions about their patients and about their shifts.

Fred knew how to mind the gap. See past your blind spot and cast light on the difference between what you intend with words and action and the impact they have on others. Fred B.'s intention was to catch up on emails and tackle problems from the moment he arrived on the unit. But his staff saw him as angry upon arrival. When he focused on the gap between his good intention and the negative impact on his staff, he was able to learn a new lesson about his leadership.

Listen to Elena V. describe how she bridged the gap between intention and impact: "When my staff are in the hall or at a computer, I don't interrupt them to say, 'Hello, how's your day going?' because they get interrupted all the time. But I discovered that my behavior was received as being someone who doesn't care. So I just talk about that now. I learned that it's possible to be misunderstood."

EXPERIMENT

Drill down to the details and shift your stance from "that's wrong" to "tell me more," advise Harvard Law professors Douglas Stone and Sheila Heen.[8] Whether you are dealing with a sneak attack in the hallway, a coaching session, or a formal performance evaluation, they suggest queries that look *backward* and forward.

Describe some recent uncomfortable feedback you have received from a colleague, team member, or supervisor. Did you get—or can you seek—the answers to the following:

What did they observe?

....

....

....

....

....

What were the criteria they used?

....

....

....

....

....

Did they specify the skills or experience that you were missing? What they were looking for? What you should be working on?

....

....

....

....

....

REFLECTION

Discover déjà vu. The bravest action—and for that reason, one of the richest sources of learning—is asking a simple and scary question: *Have I ever heard this before?* At another job? At a less-than-happy family holiday dinner? A savvy nurse manager who struggles to avoid giving mixed "yes/but" messages to her staff admits that when she explains a decision to her son, he says, "Okay, Mom, here comes the but ..."

Describe a situation when you received critical feedback that sounded uncomfortably familiar. How can seeing a pattern allow you to step up to consider changing this behavior or attitude?

....

....

....

....

....

EXPERIMENT

Don't get back on your horse. Discard the idea that you must immediately respond to criticism that throws you off balance. Create a thoughtful pause by restating what they have said. To the director who suggests that you are too controlling, you might say, "From your perspective, I micromanage my staff instead of giving them a chance to grow."

A paraphrase gives you some time to consider the comment. And, to avoid a defensive rebuttal, you can also hit pause by stating, "You have really given me a lot to think about" or "Now that I have a clear sense of what your concerns are, I will need some time to sort out what you have told me."

REFLECTION

Think again about that uncomfortable feedback. How might the advice of "not getting back on your horse" inform your response to feedback?

....

....

....

....

....

Key #4: Study Success as Carefully as Missteps

Wisdom is won in considering success stories as well as the wake-me-when-this-is-over moments. As Elaine R. instructs us, "When I look back, I say those are valuable lessons for me because that is what built me up to what I am today. You learn from small steps ... and you gather everything and put it in your notebook. When you go back and study it, you can say, 'Oh yeah, I should have done differently here or I could have been better.' Or sometimes you say, 'I'm really proud of myself that I was able to do this.'"

Learning from experiences means integrating lessons that are both imitative and corrective. When you inspire trust from your staff by apologizing for your mistakes, you learn the power of fessing up instead of covering up. Because you experienced frustration with a director with a closed-door policy, you learned the importance of being visible to your own staff. In both cases, there is a kind of inductive logic: You move from particular situation to a more general lesson of what you will to do in a similar situation in the future.

REFLECTION

Describe a time you succeeded in resolving a problem, creating innovation, or meeting a challenge. Identify the specific actions, words, and attitudes that you believe led to the positive outcome.

....

....

....

....

....

Next, describe a person whose behavior—either exemplary or dodgy—taught you a lesson you wanted to imitate or correct. How have you integrated this lesson into your practice?

....

....

....

....

....

EXPERIMENT

Establish a growth mindset. In her elegantly argued book, *Mindset*, psychologist Carol Dweck locates our capacity for persistence, resilience, and success by describing the power of a *growth mindset*—a set of beliefs grounded in the idea that effort and practice can increase your abilities.[9] She contrasts this with the static stance of a *fixed mindset*—one where you believe that your abilities and talents are established at birth.

Compare the potential of a fixed-mindset leader, who thinks, "I just can't read people. I never could," versus someone with a growth mindset, who admits, "Reading people is hard for me, but with practice and coaching I can improve."

Make a statement that describes a skill or ability in your leadership that you do not see as one of your strengths.

....

....

....

....

....

Did you describe this with a fixed mindset ("What's the use?") or one that you are approaching with effort and practice ("I am struggling, but I can practice.")? How would each of these statements affect your leadership?

....

....

....

....

....

The practice of wise leadership requires the discipline of memory.[10] It demands that you are alert to early warning signs so you avoid a wash-rinse-repeat cycle of making the same mistakes. Just listen to Nina H., who discovered that her passionate opinions telegraphed the impression that she was not listening. "I have learned to recognize my communication style when I am impassioned about something and when I was becoming irrational. When my mind is processing fast, I tend to give the impression that what you have to say is not important because I've already gotten to the solution."

"So I have two mantras that I say to myself. One is 'slow down your speech,' and the other is 'lower your voice.'"

You can use metaphors or analogies as reminders of what you have learned. Amy C. created a metaphor to remind herself of an event and her commitment. Amy was orienting a new OR nurse when she realized that she was doing everything for her instead of letting her learn on her own. It was only when Amy removed her gloves—and decided not to scrub in—that the novice nurse became confident in her practice.

Amy elaborates: "[Since then], I remind myself frequently to 'remove my gloves' when working with staff in situations where they need to address the change or issue on their own. As a manager, I am here to support and foster their growth and ideas, not to do their job for them. I have also learned that there are some decisions that need to be made by management. In those cases, *only* the manager can wear the gloves. It is just as important [to know] when to 'remove the gloves' as knowing when to keep them on."

Nina and Amy teach us that the memory of what you have learned is the wise heart of your education as a leader.

REFLECTION

Describe an essential leadership lesson you have learned—a success, a disappointment, or an unhappy surprise. What would be an analogy or metaphor that can help remind you of what you learned in that situation?

Ask a Nurse Leader: Peer Wise Ideas About Learning From Experience

Pick one or more of these examples of peer wisdom to explore.
What lessons from your own experience come to mind as you read these stories?

◇◇◇◇◇◇◇◇◇◇◇◇

"When I first started as a nurse manager, to say that I was nervous, and maybe even questioning whether I should be there, would be an understatement. On my first day in the office, as I was sitting at my desk, I had this terrible feeling that I did not belong there. I got out of my chair and just started walking around the unit. I talked to people; I laughed with them and reassured them and probably myself that we were going to be OK. I heard afterward that the staff were thrilled that I came out onto the floor to chat with them.

"From that moment forward, I made a point to start the day on the floor with staff, talking, asking questions, reminding them of our goals, and asking the nurses what they needed. Although the first day as a new manager scared me, the practice of leadership rounding is still something I do today. It is one of the best ways that I know to connect with staff and understand the needs of the unit."

Kirsten B.

Manager, Emergency Department

◇◇◇◇◇◇◇◇◇◇◇◇

"I had a nurse that I was always getting patient and family complaints about. And on this particular day, it was just one complaint too many. So I marched out on the unit (I looked to see if anyone was in the hall—which there wasn't) and I just let her have it. Stating, 'I am getting sick of getting complaints about you. This patient said you did _____ and I am just sick of it. You need to do a better job.' As I walked back to my office, I thought, 'Well, I took care of that!'

"The next day I had a full-page email from her (I called it throwup on a page). She blasted me for everything … what a terrible manager I was, showing no respect, etc. Well, that made me even angrier. I went to my mentor and said, 'I just need you to listen to me. Don't say anything.' I told her about it and read the email. I really thought she was going to agree and understand why I was so angry. Well, she said one thing to me that I will never forget: 'Did you ever get her side of the story?' The only thing I could say was 'no.'

"I went back down to my unit, went and found this nurse. I asked her if I could speak to her, either in my office or, if she preferred, an empty patient room. She chose the empty patient room. We went in, closed the door, and the first thing I did was apologize: Apologized for having the conversation in the middle of the hallway. Apologized for not getting her side of the story. She accepted my apology. I then asked her to tell me what happened. We talked it over, and how the patients and families perceive her, and what can we do to make this better. We worked on a solution together.

"What I realized later was that, by me being vulnerable as a leader and apologizing, it made my leadership stronger. This nurse and I were able to build a stronger relationship; one built on trust. I could always count on her to give me feedback and I encouraged her to do so. I was also able to have those developmental conversations with her when she needed it and a mutual respect was formed."

Beth B.
Manager, Pediatrics—Acute Care

◇◇◇◇◇◇◇◇◇◇◇

"One of my previous bosses said something to me that I have taken with me and repeated time and time again. She said, 'You can learn from watching people do it the right way, and you can learn from watching them do it the wrong way.' I have had many positive and a few negative experiences that have shaped the leader I am today. Here is one specific example:

"Over the past three years, my unit has been going through a culture transformation. The journey hasn't been easy. ... It started off up an icy hill with many challenging obstacles. However, we are finally in a great state and working on sustaining our gains. A few months ago, our organization restructured and I began reporting to a new leader. In the midst of all this change, my former boss expressed her dissatisfaction with the realignment and commented, 'After I just got you guys where I wanted you.' That single comment was one of the most deflating and insulting things I have ever had a boss say to me, especially given that she was a distant leader and in fact was responsible for some of the challenges we faced on our journey.

"While I think I did this before that experience, I am now even more apt to practice the strategy of being humble and gracious with your team's successes. Deflect the attention and praise to the boots on the ground. It will pay off for you ten-fold. There is a quote by Mary Anne Radmacher: 'As we work to create light for others, we naturally light our own way.'

Erik M.
Clinical Director, Pediatric Intensive Care Unit

◇◇◇◇◇◇◇◇◇◇◇

"When I first became the manager of a unit, I found out that the scheduling practices of the floor did not meet the need of the patients. I had to take over and do the schedule myself, change the holiday rotation, and make a shift in the weekend option staff to make sure that the unit was covered all the time.

"At first the staff was not very happy with the changes, but when they realized that the staffing was balanced and we were not short on some days and had to float or cancel on other days, the staff liked it. I feel that now the staff knows that I am going to do what is right for the patient and the staff. I also feel that now, when I come up with new items, the staff is more likely to listen and embrace any change quicker because they know I am looking at both the patient and the staff."

Melvin B.
Clinical manager

◇◇◇◇◇◇◇◇◇◇

"I had oriented a few nurses to the operating room before and it usually went well, so I followed the same plan. But in this case, I was having some difficulty with the nurse engaging in her role and I was taking on the entire responsibility during the procedure while she watched. After a few days of this, I realized that I was doing everything for her instead of letting her learn by doing. She could tell me what she should do when we reviewed the steps, she just wasn't doing it because I wasn't letting her. Ultimately, I realized that I needed to not scrub into the procedure, [but] be there to support her by communicating with her during the case and answering her questions. It only took a few cases before she was off and running on her own and very confident in her own practice.

"Today, I remind myself frequently to 'remove my gloves' when working with staff in situations where they need to address the change or issue on their own. As a manager, I am here to support and foster their growth and ideas, not to do their job for them. Through continued practice and experience in leadership, I have also learned that there are some decisions that need to be made by management. In those cases, only the manager can wear the gloves. Therefore, just as important as knowing when to 'remove the gloves' is knowing when to keep them on."

Amy N.
Manager of Care Coordination

◇◇◇◇◇◇◇◇◇◇

"I have worked as a nurse manager in two different organizations. The first one I had a great manager who helped develop me and build my confidence. I always felt she was on my team and had my best interest at heart. I learned many things from her that helped me develop into the manager that I am today. At another organization, I had a manager who was not so willing to develop me. I always felt there was competition, jealously, and the desire to see me fail. This is not a good feeling to have when you are trying to do your best. I tried through the years to ignore these thoughts and to work as 'peacefully' as I could with her. I sought out different mentors and looked for opportunities to develop myself. I took advantage of every opportunity I was given.

"As I was given these opportunities, I still always had the feeling that my manager wanted to see me fail. I didn't trust her or respect her. I didn't feel safe having this conversation with her because she was 'my boss.'

"As I continue to build my confidence and reputation by demonstrating positive outcomes, I have realized that I don't really need my boss on 'my side.' I can accomplish great things with the support of others in the organization who recognize my work. I might never get the top tier on my evaluation while under this manager, but I know that I am the top tier, and others in the organization do also. So the lesson learned, and how I practice as a manager today, is to be grateful for your staff and to help develop them every way you can. When they shine, you shine."

Carin B.
Clinical Manager

◇◇◇◇◇◇◇◇◇◇◇◇

"Here is a lesson I learned early as a leader. It was early in my role of the unit director on my current unit. I had a bad habit of entering the unit in the morning usually bothered by something I read in an email before coming on to the unit, or a leftover issue from the night before. Upon my arrival to the unit, I never took the time to ask our night shift how their shift went or if there were any issues I needed to help them with. I just began my rant.

"One day, two of our staff came to my office and looked very worried. Both were past students of mine when I was a clinical instructor. When I asked, they began to tell me how I never asked them about their shift, how things were, or anything about our shift. The day for them ended with an angry unit director on top of an already stressful shift.

"Considering the source of this information, I was taken aback. These were two very accomplished nurses. I was glad that they both valued our relationship enough to come in to give me feedback on my performance as a leader. I never forgot their message. I thanked them both for the feedback and for being brave enough to tell me I was falling short as a leader.

"Today, many, many, months later, I continue to round on the night shift, asking specific questions about their patients and about their shifts. Both nurses have transitioned to other units, but I never forget the valuable lesson they taught me about leadership. Their feedback helped shaped me into the leader I am today."

Frederick B.
Unit Director

Your Thoughts?

Describe lessons from your own experience that one or more of these stories brought to mind.

....

....

....

....

....

....

....

Q & Q: Quote and Question

Consider each quote about wisdom and answer the follow-up question from your leadership practice.

> Q: "If there's one thing I've learned over the years, it's that it only takes one person, one patient, one moment to change your life forever, to change your perspective, color your thinking. To force you to re-evaluate everything you think you know. To make you ask yourself the toughest questions: Do you know who you are? Do you know what's happened to you? Do you want to live this way?"
>
> **Dr. Christina Yang on *Grey's Anatomy***
> **(a show where doctors do the work of nurses)**

Q: Describe one person, one patient, one moment that changed your life and perspective. How do you apply what you learned in your practice?

....

....

....

....

> Q: "Science, my lad, is made up of mistakes, but they are mistakes which it is useful to make, because they lead little by little to the truth."
>
> **Jules Verne,**
> ***A Journey to the Center of the Earth***

Q: Can you describe a mistake that led you to a larger truth?

....

....

....

....

> Q: "Disappointment is the nurse of wisdom."
>
> **Sir Boyle Roche**

Q: **Describe a disappointing experience or relationship in your leadership. How did it or could it become a "nurse of wisdom" in your practice?**

....

....

....

....

> Q . "Trying to grow up is hurting. You make mistakes, you try to learn from them. When you don't, it hurts even more."
>
> **Aretha Franklin**

Q: **Describe a time when you made a mistake, did not stop to learn from it, and found yourself in the same painful situation again. What did you learn?**

....

....

....

....

> Q: "We don't live through life only by our own experiences, we live through life with other people's experience as a reference too."
>
> **Nike Thaddeus**

Q: **Describe the actions or words of another person that become a frame of reference— either an imitative or corrective lesson—for you.**

....

....

....

....

Deep Dive Resources: Wisdom of Experience

Books

American Journal of Nursing. (2017). *Reflections on nursing.* Wolter Klower.

Bion, W. R. (1991). *Learning from experience.* Jason Aronson.

Christensen, C. (2012). *How will you measure your life?* Harper Collins.

Dweck, C. (2006). *Mindset: The new psychology of success.* Ballantine.

Gutland, L. (2013). *I wasn't strong like this when I started out: Stories of becoming a nurse.* Infact Books.

Ruderman, M., & Ohlott, P. (2007). *Turning life's lessons into leadership experiences.* Center for Creative Leadership.

Stone, D.. & Heen, S. (2014). *Thanks for the feedback: The science and art of receiving feedback well.* Viking.

Thomas, R. (2008). *The crucibles of leadership: How to learn from experience to become a great leader.* Harvard Business School.

Professional Journals

Arbon, P. (2004). Understanding experience in nursing. *Journal of Clinical Nursing, 13*(2), 150–157.

Asselin, M.E., & Fain, J. A. (2013). Effect of reflective practice education on self-reflection, insight, and reflective thinking among experienced nurses: A pilot study. *Journal for Nurses in Professional Development, 29*(3), 111–119.

Horton-Deutsch, S., & Sherwood, G. (2008). Reflection: An educational strategy to develop emotionally-competent nurse leaders. *Journal of Nursing Management, 16*(8), 946–954.

Joyce, P. (2010). Leading and leadership: Reflections on a case study. *Journal of Nursing Management, 18*(4), 418–424.

Larson, D., & Brady, E. (2001). Learning stories of our own. *Adult Learning, 11*(4), 13–15.

Ramvi, E. (2015). I am only a nurse: A biographical narrative study of a nurse's self-understanding and its implication for practice. *BMC Nursing, 14*(1), 4–9.

Videos

Dweck, C. (2014, November). *The power of believing that you can improve* [Video]. TED Conferences. https://www.ted.com/talks/carol_dweck_the_power_of_believing_that_you_can_improve

Figure Credit

Motivation

Move Beyond Carrots and Sticks

"Motivation begins at home. In order to motivate the staff, the leader neeeds to be motivated. However, sometimes there is just so much to do ... it is hard to be motivated about one more thing to do."

◇◇◇◇◇◇◇◇◇◇◇◇◇◇◇◇◇◇◇◇◇

Motivation is the act of producing a reason that causes us to take action. Your colleague has underlined the twin tasks for nurse leaders—motivation of self and others. Or, as airline hosts are fond of putting it: Please put on your own oxygen mask before helping others. In this laboratory, we will explore four ways these two tasks are linked.

Motivation has always part of the core curriculum of nursing school, and you can probably describe Maslow's hierarchy of needs,[1] Skinner's pigeons pecking for positive reinforcement,[2] and the difference between carrots and sticks with your eyes closed.

But there are some new motivation teachers in town, and a new school of thinking about motivation as a kind of inner work. New school approaches suggest that external rewards—like money and prizes—though appropriate for short-term, routine tasks and team building, can trample creativity and undermine long-term performance, persistence, and engagement.

New school motivation is less about prizes and more about purpose; less about rewards and more about regard; less about answers and more about autonomy. In sum, the theory and practice of motivation is focused on inspiration rather than manipulation. It is also about keeping a line of sight to purpose.[3]

Listen to Doris E., walking into walls on a hellish day, who passed a staff nurse with her knees bent—to establish eye contact with a pediatric patient. "Watching our nurse, I realized: This is what we really do. At the end of the day, my work contributes to the person at the bedside providing the patient with excellent care. We get so busy keeping the rocks off the road that we get misaligned. That was 4 years ago, but I can still see that nurse."[4]

Because your leadership practice includes motivating yourself and your team, we begin with the idea that what motivates you may not motivate others. Doris E. was inspired by reconnecting with her pediatric patients, but she cannot assume that her team members are also energized by purpose.

Take a moment to define your theory of motivation by completing these two sentences.

I think the main thing that motivates people is ...

....

....

....

....

....

When I am feeling disengaged and unmotivated, I always ...

....

....

....

....

....

Compare the two sentences. How do these beliefs inform your practice?

....

....

....

....

....

Four Keys to Motivation as a Leadership Practice

Consider four keys to motivation as a leadership practice for yourself and others. As you read, continue to reflect on your experiences, and compare your theories of motivation with the ones that follow. Identify your best practices and plan to experiment with some new actionable strategies.

Key	Strategies	Your best practices
Key #1 Purpose	~Begin with why. ~Maintain line of sight. ~Show your thought bubble. ~Tap into team identity.	
Key #2 Regard	~Praise with specifics. ~Practice humble inquiry. ~Choose a language of appreciation.	
Key #3 Autonomy	~Promote the power of choice. ~Avoid faux feedback. ~Dare to delegate. ~Gift the next generation.	
Key #4 Mastery	~Make them authors of their accomplishments. ~Turn complaints into intentions. ~Focus on affirmative outcomes. ~Fan the flames of effort.	

Key #1: Purpose

Motivation begins and blossoms by asking why, suggests management consultant Simon Sinek.[5] Leaders know that keeping the team focused on purpose is part of the job description. Yet the challenge lies in maintaining a clear line of sight to the shared mission while you sweat the details of multiple meetings, nagging emails, insistent texts, schedule snafus, team drama, and surprise JAHCO visits.

Like Doris E., who realized "this is what we do," two wise managers offer strategies to ask and answer the why. Sharon J. explains, "I continue to drive with that force that it is [all about] the patient, the person in the bed." Tuyen K. has a created mantra for her own motivation. "I bring my best to work every day and this is what inspires me. Every day I look at me and say, whose life are you going to make better or easiest today?"[6]

The poet David Whyte defines the focus on purpose and big-picture outcomes as "the discipline of memory."[7] And Beverly L. describes her discipline during the times of inner team warfare. "If I can stay focused on the bigger picture and the broader perspective of why I was in the role and why I wanted to continue, that helps me to then not focus on the little petty things." Beverly's lesson: When you can steady your line of sight and stay focused on your purpose, you are ready to inspire team members suffering from memory loss.

REFLECTIONS

In musical composition, the word motif (based on motive) is used to describe underlying themes. Think of Beethoven's four-note opening of the Fifth Symphony that appears as a theme and variation throughout this universally adored piece. If you think of your purpose as a musical motif, what is the recurrent theme—the music—of why you do what you do?

....

....

....

....

....

EXPERIMENT

Create a word cloud about your sense of purpose. Go to https:/www. freewordcloudgenerator.com/. Follow the general instructions, and follow these prompts for your word choices:

- List five action verbs that are related to your purpose as a nurse leader (e.g., solve problems).

....

....

....

....

....

- List five nouns that are central to your purpose (e.g., coach).

....

....

....

....

....

- List five describers/adjectives that are related to your mission (e.g., supportive).

....

....

....

....

....

REFLECTIONS

What patterns and themes do you see in your word cloud that drive your sense of purpose?

....

....

....

....

....

EXPERIMENT

To discipline the memory of your team, nurse leader Eileen Magri urges you to think out loud: "Show them your thought bubble."[8] Remind them what motivates you and why; explain the bigger picture. When there are questions and resistance about a new policy, describe the facts and feelings that influenced your decision.

Get out from behind your paperwork and talk about your purpose—what you find gratifying and satisfying about your work. Motivation is contagious, so be sure to share stories that move you and motivate you, and talk about projects that excite you and the highpoint experiences that help you remember why you became a nurse.

Fill in this thought bubble with a story about your own motivation that you could pass on to your team.

IMG 2.1

EXPERIMENT

Tap into team and group identity to build meaning and motivation. Protect time in team meetings to tell patient stories or to create group statements of purpose. Have each member write a one-sentence statement of why on an index card.

The statement can be specific (Why does this goal matter?) or general (What is the purpose of our unit?). Place cards in a brown bag and read them aloud. Guide discussion around shared themes of purpose.

Key #2: Regard

Positive feedback can become the fast food of motivation. Amid your shouts of "Bravo!" "Encore!" and "Let's get pizza!" consider psychologist Robert Kegan's suggestion that a more lasting motivator is communicating regard and what he calls "the value of being valued."[9] In this approach, pizza and praise have a place on the table. But the emphasis is on what Rachel M. describes as "knowing that each individual brings something to the department and working through those gifts or challenges with each person."

Attunement to each individual requires language that is specific rather than global.[10] It also means paying attention to what my mother, Selma, a former nurse manager, called "the little things that mean a lot." For example, he has a sister undergoing chemo, her softball team won the regionals, or his son is leaving for college. It is instruction to recall the examples and models of attunement you have encountered.

REFLECTIONS

Describe an experience with a supervisor or preceptor who conveyed regard for you by listening and recognizing your gifts and challenges. What were their specific actions and statements that conveyed your value?

....

....

....

....

....

Next describe a supervisor or preceptor who told instead of asked, and whose praise was generic or rare.

....

....

....

....

....

How did your experience with each of these leaders inform your practice?

....

....

....

....

....

Attunement as a leadership practice means offering the phrase "good job" early retirement. Instead, communicate regard by being *specific* about the team member's actions, attitudes, and strengths.

EXPERIMENT

Organize your message of attunement and positive regard with this 3W formula: when—what—why it matters.

When: "This morning in our meeting."

What: "You summarized all of the frustration our team was feeling without getting everyone more upset. You showed how well you listen."

Why it matters: "When you calmly acknowledged the feelings in the room, you lowered the temperature and helped us refocus on making a good decision."

EXPERIMENT

Put this formula into your practice. Identify someone whose effort or contribution stood out to you this week. Create a 3W statement to convey to him or her.

When:

....

....

....

....

....

What:

....

....

....

....

....

Why it matters:

....

....

....

....

....

EXPERIMENT

Counselor Gary Chapman and psychologist Paul White have named five different preferences for appreciation at work.[11] They begin, as we have, with words of affirmation (praise of accomplishments, character, personality). They also suggest that each individual may seek a different expression of your appreciation. Consider each of the preferences and their match with your team members.

The other four preferences are *quality time* (focused attention, quality conversation, shared experiences), *acts of service* (offering help, pitching in, doing it their way), *tangible gifts* (thoughtful gifts the person values, time off), and *touch* (handshake, shoulder pat, high five, hug).

REFLECTION

Shame and blame are the enemies of regard. Consider this photograph/drawing. What recollections does it evoke?

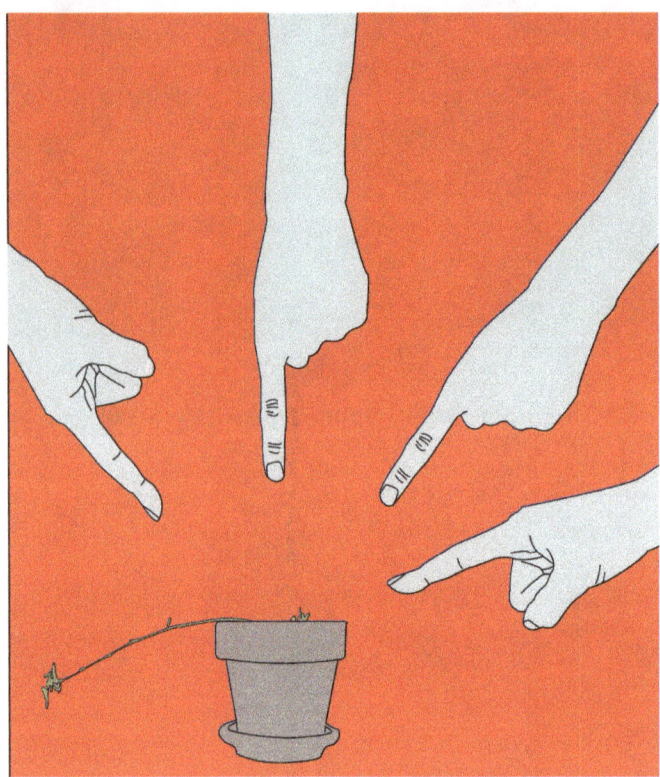

FIGURE 2.1

....

....

....

....

....

....

....

....

....

Describe a time when you were shamed or blamed. Or, when you shamed or blamed a team member. What lessons did this experience suggest for your leadership?

....

....

....

....

....

The language of regard is also anchored in the nuanced way you listen. Psychologist Edgar Schein describes a powerful practice he calls humble inquiry, which he defines as the art of asking instead of telling.[12] As he explains, "This means getting to know someone by asking questions—to which you do not know the answer—and building a relationship built on curiosity and genuine interest."

EXPERIMENT

Craft leading questions. Consider a repurposed cliché: It is a leader's lack of curiosity that will kill motivation. Adopt the approach of Ed C., who gathered the team to discuss an employee engagement survey. "We began by talking about the positive aspects of our jobs. We asked each person: What makes a great day at work for you? What does your department do well?"

Like all leaders, you get the work done through other people. For this reason, the inner homework of motivating self-regard—of being attuned to your own strengths—is your hardest assignment. It requires identifying with your team's successes and stretches, advises Cheryl M. "Seeing their world change and improve as a result of their ideas coming to fruition is as motivating for me as it is for them." It also means being specific about what you contribute to your team.

REFLECTION

Connect the dots to track your contribution to your team members' development. Describe your strengths and contributions that enable your team members to blossom.

....

....

....

....

....

Key #3: Autonomy

In Daniel Pink's sacred cow–kicking book, *Drive*, he offers an anatomy of autonomy as a motivator.[13] He is a leadership educator who urges managers to fuel autonomy and enhance a team's sense of control by empowering individuals and teams to make choices about tasks, timing, and approaches. The payoff, promises Pink, is increased staff engagement and accountability.

As a leader who encourages autonomy, honesty must be your policy. So beware of faux feedback. Don't ask your team "What would you do?" if you already know what you *plan* to do. Nothing flattens motivation more than to be asked and then told.

EXPERIMENT

....

Be clear about changes and innovations that are non-negotiable. Motivate by underlining areas where the team *can* choose: If they can't choose the *what* (You are moving to online patient charting), maybe they can choose the *when* (target date December or January), or the *who* (who might be a change champion), or the *how* (What kind of training or tutorials do they think will work best?).

The practice of generativity, the subject of Laboratory 5, is another dimension of autonomy. Psychologists Erick Erickson,[14] Dan McAdams, and Ed de St. Aubin[15] have described the pleasure leaders experience in passing on and "offering up" what they built by gifting the next generation with autonomy, power, and respect.

Leading with generativity means that you learn to motivate—and be motivated by—giving the kids the keys to the car, letting them drive with their ideas, or attend a conference in your place. It means applauding their autonomy and being excited that the unit ran smoothly during your vacation.

Beth B. describes this autonomy as a form of mutual motivation. "Empower your team to find the solution(s) and then recognize them for a job well done. This will empower them to step up again and again. It is very rewarding as a leader to see your teams become more engaged. And in the end, it can mean less work for you."

Describe a time your team came to you with a burning issue and you emboldened them to find a solution or a challenge.

....

....

....

....

....

EXPERIMENT

Dare to delegate. Raise your hand if you recognize Anna W.'s reluctance. "I would like to be able to delegate more of the day-to-day things to my charge nurses," she admitted. "But right now, they are resistant to taking on those tasks, and I find it feels quicker to just do things myself."

Successful delegation—the motivating kind that contributes to a team's sense of autonomy—begins with identifying the things that *only* you can do and then matching the appropriate person with other tasks. The *how* may be more essential than the *who*. So be clear about the purpose of the assignment, create checkpoints and benchmarks, establish the reporting relationship and the level of their authority (How much over-sight/insight will you provide? Who will make a final decision?). Delgate the outcome and not the approach. This means accepting the deliverable without the buzzkill dis-claimer of "That's not how *I* would have done it."

Key #4: Mastery

Behavioral researchers like Bernard Weiner suggest that if motivation were game of poker, mastery would trump reward.[16] Mastery resides in the sense that you are the author of your accomplishments. Weiner describes the process of attribution and suggests that the way we explain outcomes influences our beliefs and feelings about our achievements and determines our motivation and persistence in the future.

As a practical matter, this means insisting that your team members explain positive outcomes as a result of their ability and/or effortful struggle. Those who attribute their accomplishments a matter of luck or circumstance may feel less pride in their success and more shame in mistakes or failure. Calculate the mastery quotient by saying, "You showed so much self-control—you never took the bait when Mr. Wallace starting yelling," versus "You sure dodged the bullet on that one."

Toni C. calls attention to increasing mastery with the practice of appreciative inquiry, an approach created by management psychologist David Cooperrider and Suresh Srivastva[17] As she explains, "I search for the best and the good around us. I tend to focus on our positive quality outcomes, and share daily with the staff, and this seems to motivate staff more toward better outcomes. If we focus on what we are not doing right, then staff become disengaged (they feel a sense of failure) and this suffocates innovation and creativity."

REFLECTIONS

Answer two questions in quick succession.

What is my team doing wrong?

....

....

....

....

....

What is my team doing right?

....

....

....

....

Compare your motivation to meet challenges and work with your team after each answer.

....

....

....

....

....

EXPERIMENT

Guide your staff to claim their accomplishments by describing successes in terms of effort, difficulty, and ability. (Examples: "Our fall initiative was a success because you wouldn't give up and it really paid off." "It was a tall order and you filled it." "You have developed the kind of empathy that makes our patients feel less alone.")

Fine-tune mastery by rewriting complaints into statements of intention. Instead of asking what's wrong, you can ask, "What do we want more of?" Instead of allowing the team huddle to devolve into a coffee kvetch, you can inquire, "What is working?"

EXPERIMENT

Fan the flames. Identify and track masterful effortful behaviors in your team. Acknowledge and highlight their actions. For the Johnny- or Judy-come-lately who arrived on time (for once), you might say, "This morning you brought so much energy to our team meeting. It gave all of us a boost." Note to self: This can only work minus eye rolls, irony, and sarcasm.

Remember, too, that your leadership actions to build motivation may include one or more of the four keys you have explored. Consider George R., who was concerned about the disengagement of Donna M., one of the patient care technicians on his team. He decided to ask her to join a team working on a project to enhance inventory and supply of patient rooms.

He described her growing engagement. "On this team, we all view each other as equals and listen to each other's ideas, suggestions, and concerns. The respect shown by the team for Donna's knowledge on supplies, workflow, and unit needs have motivated her to take on increased ownership within the unit."

An anatomy of George's approach reveals all four keys of motivation: By appointing Donna to this project group at a time of her diminished motivation, he conveyed his regard for her expertise and emboldened her to offer the knowledge of her lived experiences. The project also provided Donna with the opportunity to display her mastery and to nurture her renewed sense of purpose.

As you continue to build a vibrant community of practice, take note of your successes in motivating yourself and your team. What are the gestures, attitudes, and actions that were the catalysts of your (or their) increased engagement and investment of time and talent?

Ask a Nurse Leader: Peer Wise Ideas About Motivation

Pick one or more of these examples of peer wisdom to explore.
What lessons from your own experience come to mind as you read these stories?

◇◇◇◇◇◇◇◇◇◇◇

"Motivation must come from within a person. I feel it is impossible to motivate someone without his or her participation. I motivate myself by reading and learning best practices and sharing ideas with leaders from across various organizations outside of health care. I use that knowledge to create new ideas and new approaches to face challenges ahead.

"I also believe taking care of oneself (for me, through yoga and exercise) is essential to ensuring you have the energy to sustain motivation of yourself, which in turn inspires others. I motivate staff that has natural talents and abilities by sharing my observations with them about the things they are really great at. A focus on the positive nurtures your team and increases their own motivation to do more and be more."

Kelly B.

Administrative Director, Service Excellence

◇◇◇◇◇◇◇◇◇◇◇

"You need to work for an organization with nursing leaders who support your innovation and creativity. The support for working with staff to use small tests of change to improve the working environment on the unit by your immediate supervisor is crucial to both your credibility and success as a leader. Asking the question of your staff ('What would you do?') stimulates critical thinking for problem solving and inspires leadership qualities to evolve. Don't settle for the 'status quo'; reflect on what is working along with what is not working and collaborate with staff for improvement. Try to anticipate what the next change will be and prepare the staff to adjust. Don't be afraid to take a risk.

"Get involved in professional activities, whether it be involvement in your specialty organization, a presentation, or publishing. This serves as a model to your staff and you can then develop and mentor your staff.

"I would have to say that my motivation for igniting the passion to continue in the role of nurse manager is the challenge my nurse director and CNO gives me to explore new opportunities for the advancement of my involvement in unit, hospital-wide initiatives, and personal professional growth through her support of my involvement in AONE [American Organization of Nursing Leaders] and other professional activities."

Susanne Y.

Manager, Surgery and Neuro-Trauma

◇◇◇◇◇◇◇◇◇◇◇

"The nurse manager role is the toughest job in my opinion. It can be emotionally exhausting. The rewards can sometimes be hidden and you need to search for them. Remember on your most difficult days that you make a difference. It is easy to forget that when dealing with challenging patients and staff. Find what your staff is passionate about; help them realize the positive impacts they can make. When staff feels empowered to make change, then they will be motivated at work. Tell them they make a difference; reward them for going above and beyond. Show your staff that you are invested in them and care about them. It will create a healthy work environment and foster a team atmosphere."

Tara M.

Manager, Adolescent Unit

"I learned through the AONL Nurse Manager Leadership training in 2012 about evidence-based practice around appreciative inquiry. I tend to focus on our positive quality outcomes, and share daily with the staff. This seems to motivate our staff more toward better outcomes. If we focus on what we are not doing right, then staff become disengaged; this suffocates innovation and creativity. Staff take this personally and feel a sense of failure. Searching for the best and the good around us allows the staff and myself to focus on the positive. What we put emphasis on becomes our reality. Asking questions influences the staff to be imaginative. This is motivation … toward excellent outcomes."

Toni C.

Manager, Clinical Operations, Neuro-Trauma

"I enjoy new challenges, especially those that involve brainstorming and collaboration. So getting involved in new initiatives motivates me to keep on going. I believe strongly in shared governance and staff involvement. I set the expectation that all staff must be involved in some way on the unit, either with data collection or committees. I support them in whatever they are interested in and help them develop stretch goals and leadership opportunities. It is important to capitalize on staff strengths and steer them toward projects that interest them. The staff are so creative. Supporting them with their ideas is incredibly empowering. Seeing their world change and improve as a result of their ideas coming to fruition is as motivating for me as it is for them. It's what I enjoy most about my role as a nurse manager."

Cheryl M.

Manager, Intensive Care Unit

"I think this comes easy for me primarily because I love my job. I love what I do for my staff and patients and am willing to do what it takes to make them happy. I really focus on fun a lot at work, which, in my mind, helps with self-motivation for staff. One thing I started about 6 months ago is a monthly newsletter strictly for my departments, entitled 'The CPRN Perspective' (C-Clinical Transition Unit, P-PICC Team, R-Resource Staff, N-Nurse Admins).

It focuses on 75% fun, such as vacation photos, local events employees have attended, who kids are graduating, who just got their BSN, etc. The other 25% is business, such as education reminders, hospital news, etc.

"We also established bi-annual volunteer activities to focus on our community pillar. The last volunteer outing we did was a free spay/neuter clinic for cats and dogs. Lastly, we started having social outings for all staff, which are held on the last Friday of every quarter. Sometimes we meet at a restaurant or bar/grill and sometimes we make it a family event and have a big BBQ.

"I firmly believe having happy employees has kept them engaged with hospital initiatives and expectations."

Morgan T.
Manager, Clinical Transition Unit

◇◇◇◇◇◇◇◇◇◇◇◇

"Never give up, keep trying, because the time you make a difference in a patient's life, a staff member's life, or you see how far a person you invested in has grown for the positive, you will never question the hard work and heartache again. It is always worth it in the end!"

Tammy S.
Manager, Surgical Specialty Unit

◇◇◇◇◇◇◇◇◇◇◇◇

"One of the things that motivates me the most is when I get recognition for my staff. When I get one of my nurses being recognized for a Daisy award, employee of the month, or a big promotion, I know that my leadership and encouragement has been meaningful. I am so proud of them and the work that they do; it really motivates me to see their potential.

"What motivates members of my team? Empathy! I find that all they need sometimes is for me to listen. When I make myself available and spend the time with them, I feel like it shows that we are one team and it motivates them to do extraordinary things."

Desi S.
Manager, MCU/PCU

◇◇◇◇◇◇◇◇◇◇◇◇

"Spend time with the team identifying a common vision. Ask your staff what the perfect unit/work environment/workflow/relationship with another department looks like. Find out what aspects of the topic you're trying to motivate them about is most important to them, you, the organization, and other stakeholders to the best of your ability. Make sure they're clear that the perfect anything is most likely unattainable, but that you're committed to working with them toward the vision. If it's something you need them to do, ask them how they think they can get it done, and then listen to them.

"Every time your team accomplishes something toward the vision, brag like crazy about it. Send emails up the chain that recognize the team to their skip-level leaders, and then forward that leader's response back to them if they're not directly on the email. Print them and post them on the unit. If their performance is being measured against other units, post their rank where they can see it and track it over time. Give them the answers—don't make them struggle to know the right thing to do. If they're stuck, find out what resources are out there to help them."

Michelle K.
Manager, Emergency Community Operations/Critical Care

◇◇◇◇◇◇◇◇◇◇◇

"Think outside the box. ... Many times in health care we like to do the same thing over and over again. Look at how other companies, like Google or Zappos, engage their employees, then tweak it to fit health care. The way I motivate myself is from my managers, when they come to me with a great idea and I can break down the barriers to make them successful."

Gretchen P.
Director of Surgical Services

"Empowerment and recognition are top priority. Empower your team to find the solution(s) and then recognize them for a job well done. This will empower them to step up again and again. It is very rewarding as a leader to see your team become more and more engaged. And in the end, it can mean less work for you.

"I have had many people ask me if I miss the bedside. My reply is this: No, I still connect with the patients and families on my leadership rounds, and what I used to once give to my patients, I now give to my staff."

Beth B.
RN Manager, Pediatrics—Acute Care

◇◇◇◇◇◇◇◇◇◇◇

"I read a lot of articles on leadership to motivate and inspire myself to remain positive. I let go of things that I cannot control or have passed. All members of the team have to have equal commitment or resentments develop. All team members need to commit to the 'team plan' and vow to hold up their part of the bargain. An open atmosphere needs to be established so that all members of the team can speak openly about what's not working. Teams need to be able to have 'reset conversations,' which get the team back on track."

Steven T.
Manager, ICU/ISCU/Life Safety

◇◇◇◇◇◇◇◇◇◇◇

"Find what is important to you and then create goals around that important thing. Also, make it fun and silly. I think if we allowed more 'fun' at work we would see outcomes change. By integrating more fun at work, I mean the following. Hospitals tend to be very stoic and tradition-based organizations. I think if we took lessons from other industries, such as Southwest Airlines, Zappos, or FedEx, who built their companies around customer satisfaction … All of the companies I just mentioned (and they are all quite successful) give the employees permission to 'delight' the customer. Southwest has rapping flight attendants and FedEx has FedEx days where employees compete with each other to get pet projects resourced.

"Could you imagine the change in outcomes if a group of nurses, or better, an interdisciplinary team, wrote a rap to a special patient and then performed it for the patient? What would that do for the patient? What would that do for team spirit and camaraderie on a nursing unit? If hospital executives set the strategic plan for the organization, and then created an environment through fun and friendly competition, where certain projects were allocated resources.

"Of course, the above are bigger, grander ideas that require buy-in from the most senior levels of an organization. At my workplace, people seem to have forgotten how to have fun at work. It can be as simple as unit competitions that have no patient falls for a month, or a funny award given out to a staff member. My husband's company had a life-size cutout of John Travolta (*Saturday Night Fever* era) that they would pass to the employee of the week. It brought a sense of lighthearted fun to work. The ideas are limitless, but we have to get comfortable with having fun. Think of Patch Adams; he brought humor to healing and to hospitals. I think we just need to unbutton the top button a little and let loose."

Corrin S.
Director, Cancer Medicine Service

◇◇◇◇◇◇◇◇◇◇◇

"Always look for ways to improve ourselves as a team and individuals. Take time to celebrate the victories and always have a goal we are reaching to achieve. I am motivated by my staff. When they do amazing things, I want to match their level of excellence!"

Jill G.
Manager, Heart and Vascular ICU

◇◇◇◇◇◇◇◇◇◇◇

"I find that what motivates me is service recovery. I find that it really connects me to the patient and patient care. When I am trying to problem solve for them, I am reminded that it is for the patient and it gives me purpose. I find that if I am involved in patient care, even if it is peripherally, it fills my cup again.

"I get to connect, share, and really empathize. When I have even brief moments that I get to be 'frontline' it reminds me why I chose nursing and all of the good I can do in the role that I am in. I motivate members of my team by telling a patient story and connecting it to what we do. Having a passion for caring for patients and expressing it to my team helps them also find meaning in what they do. I also find it very motivating to hold the team (especially the high producers) accountable."

Chris A.
Manager, Medical Oncology

Your Thoughts?

Pick one or more of these examples of peer wisdom about motivation to explore. What lessons from your own experiences come to mind as you read these stories?

....

....

....

....

....

....

....

....

....

....

....

....

....

....

....

....

....

....

....

Q & Q: Quote and Question

Consider each quote about motivation and answer the follow-up question in light of your experiences.

> Q: "If a nurse can hold a dying patient and sit with a distraught family on one day, and then return to do it the next day, is there any doubt this is a motivated person? It is the unintentional de-motivation of nurses we need to worry about."
>
> **Quint Studer**

Q: **What would you include on your list of factors that "de-motivate" nurses?**

....

....

....

....

> Q. "If you hear a voice within you say you cannot paint, then by all means paint and that voice will be silenced."
>
> **Vincent van Gogh**

Q: **How do you motivate yourself when you have lost confidence or momentum?**

....

....

....

....

> Q: "Treat people as if they were what they should be and you help them become what they are capable of becoming."
>
> **Johann Von Goethe**

Q: **Can you think of an example in your own leadership that demonstrates—or refutes—this idea about motivation?**

....

....

....

....

> Q. "There are no two words in the English language more harmful than 'good job.'"
> **Terence Fletcher in** *Whiplash*

Q: **Do you agree? Explore this idea in terms of your experiences in motivating your team.**

....

....

....

....

 # Deep Dive Resources: Motivation

Books

Chapman, G., & White, P. (2019). *The 5 languages of appreciation in the workplace: Empowering organizations by encouraging people.* Northfield Publishing.

Deci, E., & Flaste, R. (1996). *Why we do what we do: Understanding self-motivation.* Penguin.

Hillard, P., & Lopez, D. (2019). *Lead, motivate. engage.* People Performance Publishing.

Pink, D. (2009). *Drive: The surprising truth about what motivates us.* Riverhead Books.

Sinek, S. (2009). *Start with why.* Penguin.

Tye, J. (2014). *The Florence prescription: From accountability to ownership.* Values Coach, Inc.

Weinschenck, S. (2013). *How to get people to do stuff.* Pearson.

Professional Journals

Atchison, T. A. (2003). Exposing the myths of employee satisfaction. *Healthcare Executive, 17*(3), 20–21.

Buckingham, M. (2005, March). What great managers do. *Harvard Business Review, 3*(3), 70–79.

Curtis, E., & O'Connell, R. (2011). Essential leadership skills for motivating and developing staff. *Journal of Nursing Management, 18*(5), 32–35.

Dunn, D. (2015). Motivation: What makes you tick? *OR Nurse*, *9*(2), 8–47.

Loke, J. (2001). Leadership behaviors: Effects on job satisfaction, productivity and organizational commitment. *Journal of Nursing Management*, *9*(4), 191–204.

Perreira, T., & Innis, J. (2016). Work motivation in health care: A scoping literature review. *International Journal of Evidence-Based Healthcare*, *14*(4), 175–182.

Toode, K., Routasalo, P., & Suominen, T. (2011). Work motivation of nurses: A literature review. *International Journal of Nursing Studies*, *48*(2), 246–257.

Videos

Cleveland Clinic. (2013, February 27). *Empathy: The human connection to patient care* [Video]. YouTube. www.youtube.com/embed/cDDWvj_q-o8

A video that captures the heart and soul of purpose in health care.

Nurse Bass. (2015, May 10). *Motivation and inspiration for nurses and nursing students* [Video]. YouTube. https://www.youtube.com/watch?v=urf3qrp1S5U

Nurse Bradley Bass offers motivation and inspiration for nurses.

RSA Animate. (2010, April 1). *Drive: The surprising truth about what motivates us* [Video]. YouTube. http://youtu.be/u6XAPnuFjJc

An animated lecture about motivation with Daniel Pink, author of *Drive*.

Figure Credit

Boundary Clarity

Maintain Perspectives and Limits

"I was a nurse for 15 years on this unit. Those staff members that were my friends were no longer. To succeed as a manager, you must be consistent and fair and do what is right for your patient … but I realize that you do have to separate yourself a little bit from the staff in order to make unbiased judgments and to make calls that are correct. You can't just be one of their buddies."

◇◇◇◇◇◇◇◇◇◇◇◇◇◇◇◇◇◇

For many nurse leaders, the need to build clear boundaries begins on the first day on the job: Tuesday you were complaining about the boss, and on Friday you *became* the boss. In this laboratory, we will explore what your colleague means when she says, "You have to separate yourself." She is describing the essence of the leadership practice of creating boundary clarity—building strong connections to others without losing your sense of self or authority.[1]

Whether you are a new manager making the transition from nurse peer to nurse leader, or a seasoned sage, you know that boundaries are those invisible lines of separation that allow you to define and shape limits and responsibilities in your relationships with staff, colleagues, physicians, patients, and families.[2]

With appropriate boundaries, you can establish and communicate what is acceptable to you and what to expect from you. Clear boundaries underline your sense of responsibility—which tasks, feelings, and outcomes belong to you and which do not. This allows you to choose how you respond to the demands and feelings of others.

By contrast, when boundaries are unclear, you can overreact and disappear into the feelings and actions of others. Your decisions are then driven by fear of someone's anger or rejection, by the desire to avoid hurting them, or being hurt or by the impulse to fix everything to protect them.[3]

Jeanette M. explains her discovery of the difference: "I needed to, when things were happening, to step back and say, 'They're not doing this to me. This is for whatever reason they've chosen to present this way, to act this way. I can't take it personally.' It was really upsetting to me at first, and then I realized I needed to stop and take a moment and realize that whatever they needed to do was their own issue and not directly related to me."

This "stepping back" is the blueprint for what social psychologist Jane Adams calls boundary intelligence. When you choose your response to others, you can also control your time and energy, which, in turn, allows you to focus on your priorities.[4]

The Boundary Crashers

Boundary clarity is a contact sport. Your boundaries are like invisible shields; they are most often revealed when someone crashes into them. Consider eight boundary crashers. With your permission, they can break down the appropriate limits you have set.

REFLECTION

Study each of the boundary crashers below and link them to your own experiences. Make note of your best practices in setting limits with each of them.

Crasher	Tactics	Catchphrase	Best practices
Mount Vesuvius	Erupts with anger, accusations, and shame	"This is your fault."	
The Procrastinator	Tries to make their emergency your emergency	"I just didn't get to this: Can you finish it for me?"	
The Confider	Gives too much information about their private life	"You are the only one I can tell this to."	
The Reporter	Asks for too much information about your private life	"Are you dating anyone?"	
The Dumpster	Frequently unloads tears and fears	"I just can't take it anymore."	
The Triangulator	Pulls you into their conflict with others	"Do you know what Tim said to me?"	
The Home Wrecker	Intrudes on your life away from work	"I'll call you at home tonight."	
The Monopolizer	Asks for more than their share of time, energy, and attention	"Got a minute?" "Just one more thing …"	

EXPERIMENT

Use your feelings of resentment or anxiety as radar to alert you to the presence of a boundary crasher, and to take steps to separate your emotional responses from theirs.

REFLECTION

Psychology educators Jan Black and Greg Enns have suggested that boundaries are a life-enhancing system of yeses and nos. They serve as signs and borders to protect yourself from people and situations that are not in your best interest.[5]

Working with this definition, describe a situation where you said yes or no—and created a boundary to protect yourself and enhance your leadership.

....

....

....

....

....

Four Keys to Enhance Boundary Clarity in Leadership

Explore four keys to enhance boundary clarity in your leadership. As you read, reflect on your experiences, add your best practices, and plan to experiment with some new actionable strategies.

Key	Strategies	Your best practices
Key #1 Accept your authority.	~Defend against boundary crashers. ~Clarify expectations. ~Avoid the pitfalls of pleasing.	
Key #2 Build thick borders.	~Maintain equilibrium. ~Step out of the triangle. ~Coach for conflict.	
Key #3 Create emotional insulation.	~Focus on facts. ~Listen to understand. ~Call time-out during tirades. ~Consider accountability.	
Key #4 Disengage to gain perspective.	~Get up on the balcony. ~Use stopping statements. ~Come home from work. ~Edit your story. ~Teach people how to treat you.	

Key #1: Accept Your Authority

Boundary clarity provides the inner authority that allows you to lead without being a buddy or a bully—to be friendly without the close friendships with your team members that can compromise your leadership. It begins when you accept that you are in charge of directing care and patient outcomes.

Taking the lead requires that you communicate your standards and expectations. This includes being clear about job responsibilities, reporting relationships, priorities, and timelines. It also means that you set informed limits with your own supervisor. And it might mean that you think twice about who can view your happy dance on Instagram or TikTok.

The acceptance of your authority requires finding the sweet spot between responding to the demands of others and taking your own needs into account. Be alert to the boundary blurring behavior of looking to be liked—which leads to trying to please all of the team, all of the time. Above all, remember that even the most enlightened authority cannot make every camper happy.

Listen to Anne D. about the pitfalls of pleasing in drafting the staff schedule: "Despite discussions and emails explaining the needs of the unit, the schedule still comes back with many requests and many days understaffed. Then I wind up having to take away requests or contacting staff to see whose request is more important. It takes so much of my time. I want to make everyone happy, but it is making me miserable."

REFLECTION

Describe a situation when you felt comfortable in accepting your authority.

....

....

....

....

....

Next, describe an experience where your desire to be a buddy, or please the crowd, crossed the boundary of your authority.

....

....

....

....

....

What would you want to teach other leaders about what you have learned?

....

....

....

....

....

REFLECTION

Respond to each of these crucial questions.
What are the rewards and necessary losses of taking charge?

....

....

....

....

....

Why am I trying so hard to make everyone happy?

....

....

....

....

....

What are the consequences of saying yes to every demand of my supervisor?

....

....

....

....

....

EXPERIMENT

Don't just say no. Employ your authority to enhance team autonomy. Try the No + Why + How formula. ("No, we can't postpone the date of switching to bedside reporting because the whole center is making the change on that date. How do you think we can best prepare for this?")

EXPERIMENT

Convey your approachability and limits with a "yes and" statement. Say to your team, "*Yes,* I can talk now *and* in ten minutes I have to take a conference call. With your supervisor: "*Yes,* I can work on the presentation *and* this means I will have to set aside the budget projections for a couple of days."

REFLECTION

Leaders can experience a sense of loss in separating from team members to establish their authority.[6] This requires cultivating trusted on-the-job colleagues and friends outside of work.

Who are the on-the-job colleagues you can confide in or seek counsel from?

....

....

....

....

....

Who are the supportive friends outside of work (people with whom you don't need to do any impression management) who you can tell the real story of your challenges as a leader?

....

....

....

....

....

Key #2: Build Thick Borders

Psychologist Edward Hartmann used the term "thick boundaries" to characterize those who are able to maintain their focus and equilibrium in the face of the strong feelings of others.[7] As Derrick L. explains, "There is a gap of the intensity that isn't mine personally, it belongs to my staff. Being able to translate that, and be an ambassador of sorts, means that I need to be able to communicate effectively."

Maintaining healthy, thick boundaries also means fencing in your own intense feelings: In one leader's memorable words, "If they see that my hair is on fire, their hair will be on fire."

Being a communication ambassador—with a fireproof hairdo—can be challenging. This can mean accepting the gripes of wrath about new procedures, refusing to take sides with the staffer feuding with the CNA or responding with a kind firmness to the son whose stinging criticism of his father's care is an expression of his own fear and grief.

REFLECTION

Recall a situation when you were able to maintain your emotional equilibrium—while others were losing theirs.

....

....

....

....

....

Next, describe an experience where the strong feelings of others erased or smudged your boundary lines.

....

....

....

....

....

Compare the outcome of the two situations.

....

....

....

....

....

Creating thicker borders also requires learning to step out of the triangle. Psychologists, such as Murray Bowen, have outlined the peril of triangulation.[8] Simply put, this refers to the all-too-frequent situation when two (or more) people in conflict try to enlist you to take sides or to rescue them. Jenna C. detailed the problem, and her straightforward solution: "I am often challenged with the conflict of empowering staff to address their peers with issues or frustrations. I often find myself listening to staff complain that 'he' is lazy or 'she' doesn't complete orders. They will complain to me and I feel as though the message would have more gravity if it was peer to peer."

She avoids triangulation by "encouraging staff to address their peers. I give them communication ideas on how to do so. I feel like the team can be stronger if everyone is accountable and works together."

Another leader explains what is at stake. He asks, "If the team are not able to settle a conflict among themselves, then how can they help patients and families work through the struggles of new or chronic medical conditions?"

EXPERIMENT

Step out of the triangle by encouraging teammates in conflict to speak directly to each other. Begin by listening and paraphrasing their concern. ("So you feel that Tim leaves orders undone.") Once you have acknowledged their concerns, redirect them to communicate one on one. ("Have you talked to Tim about it?") If they demur ("Oh, I couldn't."), coach and rehearse an approach with them. Set a date to check back in with them.

EXPERIMENT

Coach for conflict. When you direct the rehearsal for a peer-to-peer conversation, suggest guiding ground rules. One could be to avoid global attacks and pouncing on their personal traits ("you never," "you always," "you are not a team player"). Who would admit to any of those full-frontal attacks? Skip the sticky guilt and the empty threats. ("You made me cry." "If you ever do that again ...")

Instead, encourage them to focus on a specific time and behavior. ("This morning, in our meeting, you sighed and rolled your eyes when I was explaining the new rounding policy.") State how the eye roll affected you. ("I felt frustrated because I am trying to get all of our managers on board.") And finally, coach them ask for what they want the other person to start doing or stop doing. ("If you have concerns about the rounding policy, I would like you to talk to me directly.")

Key #3: Create Emotional Insulation

Thick boundaries can be fortified by creating what psychiatrist Louis Ormond calls a healthy insulation barrier.[9] This barrier is a mental boundary that allows experience in, but protects you from being overwhelmed by the negative emotions of others. It means, for example, that you understand that a nurse is not angry with you; he is upset about working on Thanksgiving.

For Julianne P., creating an insulation barrier was the crucible for remaining in the leadership role. "If I took every negative thing people had to say about the units or what's going on as an attack on me, I would have never survived."

Emotional insulation can allow you to weather both hot and cold interactions. This requires the discipline of keeping your boundaries clean and clear by imagining the other person's point of view and focusing on the facts of the situation. In doing so, you can refrain from hearing their words as rejection or stinging criticism. You can make room for understanding and problem resolution.

REFLECTION

Describe an experience when you were able to protect or insulate yourself while listening to the strong emotional responses of a staff member, colleague, physician, or patient.

....

....

....

....

....

Next, describe an experience where you felt overwhelmed by forceful words or feelings.

....

....

....

....

Compare your capacity for resolving the problem at the center of each example.

....

....

....

....

....

EXPERIMENT

Call an inner time-out when listening to a tirade. Imagine that you are speaking with a physician who is furious that one of your RNs asked her to speak with a patient for the second time that day.

Instead of preparing a defense, focus your awareness on trying to summarize her frame of reference. This is a strategy leadership educator Steven Covey describes as listening to understand rather than to reply.[10]

Acknowledge her perspective, saying, for example, "Your day is so packed and you feel like you have already spent so much time with Mrs. H." Then steer her back to the facts: "So let's figure out why Mrs. H. is having such a difficult time understanding the reason she needs to take so many medications after her surgery."

EXPERIMENT

Consider accountability. When a colleague comes charging at you, accusing you of being unfair, take a moment to erect an internal shield by considering two questions: Is there any truth about my actions in this accusation? How much of this is about the other person's feelings?

Key #4: Disengage to Gain Perspective

Leadership scholars Marty Linsky and Ronald Heifetz use the expression "getting off the dance floor and up on the balcony" to describe the boundary that is created by disengaging from heated situations in order to review the problem.[11]

Your capacity to maintain boundaries by standing back to assess problems can be enhanced by creating a pause in the conversation, a break in the action, or by refusing to work late in order to ensure a good night's sleep.

Elgin V. creates boundaries by changing location. "There are times when family members are just adamant. What I try to do is bring them into my office and remove them away from the audience and see what the real problem is. Nine times out of ten it has nothing to do with whatever they are screaming about."

REFLECTION

Describe a time when you restored your perspective by disengaging from a heated situation (i.e., you went up to your mental balcony—creating distance).

....

....

....

....

....

Next, describe an experience where you stayed too long on the dance floor.

....

....

....

....

....

How did these experiences affect your leadership practice?

....

....

....

....

....

EXPERIMENT

Abandon the idea that you have to respond immediately to every heated situation. Use statements to stop or pause a discussion. Try these stopping statements: "This is important to you and I don't want to respond too quickly." "You have really given me a lot think about." "I have a clear sense of what is bothering you; give me some time to sort out what you have told me."

EXPERIMENT

Learn how to come home from work and protect your private time—without compromising your competence. Communicate a clear policy about when (and if) you can be called at home or on vacation. Reduce your rapid response time to non-emergency, after-hours emails. When you can leave the hospital behind, you can return with a fresh perspective about unfinished business.

REFLECTION

Study this painting by Sally Deng. What feelings and insights about creating work/home boundaries does it evoke?

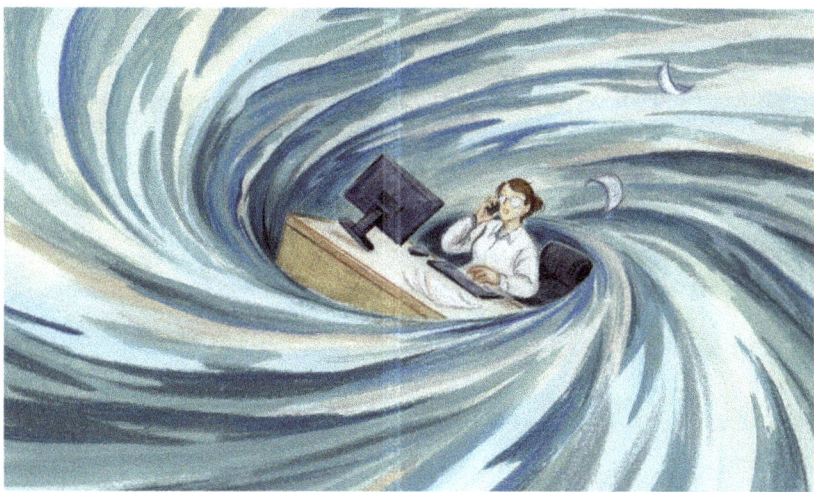

FIGURE 3.1

....

....

....

....

....

Psychologist Martin Seligman has drawn our attention to explanatory models—the stories we tell ourselves about events and relationships.[12] We all recognize three bestselling stories about boundary crashers: victim ("It is not my fault."), villain ("She made me cry."), and helpless ("There is nothing I can do.").

Boundary clarity requires that you rewrite the roles of victim and villain and exchange a sense of mastery for helplessness. Consider Ella T.'s brilliant revision of a victim/villain story—one where she invested three months supporting a staff member who then left the unit.

As she tells it, "At first, I thought, 'How dare you do that to me? I have really gone out of my way for you.' This was probably not the correct response. But I think I taught myself that she didn't do this *to me.* If I choose to react this way to it, that's my issue. I *chose* to bend over backwards for her."

And then she wrote a new role for mastery in her future. "So I had to make sure that I only give what I think is acceptable and not expect allegiance forever and forever. I can only do things that are in my control. I can't control someone else's behavior."

REFLECTION

Describe a challenging situation or relationship that compromised your boundary clarity—one that you understood in terms of you being helpless—the "victim" of a "villain."

....

....

....

....

....

First, rewrite your role from victim to actor. Consider: What is my participation in the problem? How might the other person see my role in the situation?

....

....

....

....

....

Next, rewrite the villain into a person. Consider: What is another explanation for their behavior? Can I find something positive to work with? Can I find common ground?

....

....

....

....

And finally, change your view of yourself from helpless to capable. You can shape your concern into an intention: What do I want more of? What is the long view and big picture? What is one action I can take to change the situation?

EXPERIMENT

Practice statements of mastery that allow you to respond to the demands of complicated relationships and enhance your capacity for understanding.

For example, "I can sort out which strong feelings belong to him and which to me." "I can't change or control her; I can only take charge of my response to her." "I am not responsible for his attitude or happiness, and he not responsible for mine."

Statements of boundary mastery must also include what poet Maya Angelou called "teaching people how to treat you."[13] Tina offers the example of a provider—who was running behind—yelling and throwing a stack of papers at her. She calmly replied, "You will not yell at me and I am not picking those papers up. I will be in your office to discuss your concerns and help develop solutions when you're ready."

Consider, finally, Stacy L.'s description of how the practice of boundary clarity can underline your integrity and intentions. "I better not do any more than what I *want* to do. Because that puts me in the arena of expecting something back for it. I will do it because it makes sense or it's the right thing to do." Her words suggest how boundaries can become a compass and conscience at the heart of your leadership.

Ask a Nurse Leader: Peer Wise Ideas About Boundaries

Pick one or more of these examples of peer wisdom about boundaries to explore. What lessons from your own experience come to mind as you read these stories?

◇◇◇◇◇◇◇◇◇◇◇

"The best advice I can offer is to keep boundaries between social and professional interaction when dealing with staff. I think it's important that they don't see you as their friend but as their coach or mentor.

"I would also say that a manager needs to be the calm amid the storm. Health care environments can be very emotionally charged places, but the manager needs to be the person that keeps a level head. This does not mean a manager is a pushover, but brings the team back to the reason why all of us are in health care—the patient."

Gretchen P.
Director of Surgical Services

◇◇◇◇◇◇◇◇◇◇◇

"Managers need to have a high level of emotional intelligence. I regularly practice self-reflection. I use my car ride home as my personal therapy session, where I relive the events of the day. I am able to be critical of myself and call myself out on things that I could have done better. If you are always having conflicts with others you need to be able to ask yourself, 'Maybe it's me?'

"In addition to self-awareness, a manager needs to be able to self-manage their behaviors so that they don't behave recklessly. In other words, don't take the bait! It's important to do some thinking in advance of interactions that may be volatile. Ask yourself, what do I want the outcome of this exchange to be? Stay true to that answer and remain in control."

Steven J.
Manager, ICU/ISCU

◇◇◇◇◇◇◇◇◇◇◇

"I believe you have to start with protecting your calendar. I block off time for rounds on the unit and no one can move them unless I say it is okay. Those rounds are when I touch base with staff, patients, families, etc.

"I believe that if someone is trying to impede my personal boundary, I have to let him or her know in the moment. I believe giving *and receiving* feedback is a necessity in leadership and it is best in the moment that it is happening.

"If you cannot do it right in the moment because your emotions are too high (or theirs are), then you let them know that you need to talk to them at greater length and would like to get back together to discuss. Then set up a time to do that. This gives you and them time to cool down and think rationally. I also believe that setting up expectations ahead of time or up front might avoid some of this. As leaders, we will always have 'fires' to put out, but we deal with them as they come. They typically don't come every day."

Beth B.
Manager, Pediatrics—Acute Care

◇◇◇◇◇◇◇◇◇◇

"Our unit is intense and I like to keep the atmosphere informal and open. I do share some details about my home life and take an interest in what is happening with staff members' lives, but I avoid becoming their counselor and confidant. I enjoy socializing with staff at work events once or twice a year, but otherwise do not go out with the group after work. I do not accept Facebook friend requests from staff—that is my most concrete boundary."

Cheryl M.
Manager, ICU

◇◇◇◇◇◇◇◇◇◇

"When I first became a manager, I made the decision to never give my personal home phone number or cell phone to my staff. I always carried a pager and told them if they need to have access to me they could do that via the pager. As we have become a more tech-oriented society, I see so many nurse managers giving their staff their personal cell phone numbers and texting the staff back and forth. To me this limits the staff's ability to learn problem-solving skills and reinforces with them that you are Mama Manager.

"Along those same lines, do not friend your staff on Facebook or follow them on Twitter. Some people do not practice good judgment with the things they post or tweet; as a supervisor of people, I don't want to know those details of your life, nor do I want you to know them about me. The last thing, I try and practice respect around times I call a staff member at home and respecting their time at home. I feel it is important for everyone to unplug from work so they can function at their fullest. I expect my staff to respect my time away from work; therefore, I try to return the same courtesy."

Corrin S.
Director, Cancer Medicine

◇◇◇◇◇◇◇◇◇◇

"I am a person that has been very good about keeping my emotions out of any decisions that I have to make. I feel that I have to work on showing some emotions at times. For instance, I am a person to walk into a room and start saying whatever items that I need accomplished without saying hello or asking how the staff is doing.

"So I purposefully stop myself, to make sure I ask how the staff is doing and what I can do for them, before I start with whatever I need. I try to be as honest as I can with the staff, physicians, supervisors, and patients. This lets everyone know what you think of a situation and if it needs to be addressed."

Melvin B.
Clinical manager

◇◇◇◇◇◇◇◇◇◇◇

"Empowering my nurses to be leaders in my absence. To do this, I need to give them the tools to make leadership decisions. I tell them the decision they make will always be the right one. And then I need to support them in that decision. It may not have been the decision I would have made, and sometimes it is a better decision! I try to follow up to discuss with them and give positive feedback after the fact."

Jill G.

Manager, Heart and Vascular ICU

◇◇◇◇◇◇◇◇◇◇◇

"I believe that a nurse manager needs to possess a great deal of empathy and remain relatable to staff. The conversation needs to be focused on the staff, patient, physician, and not on the self. You need to understand how they feel and the reason for the emotion they are feeling. At that point you can provide honest and compassionate feedback. I believe you must consistently be fair, honest, and unwavering in your own personal integrity, serving as a role model and getting really comfortable saying 'I'm sorry.' Always remember this is their experience."

Kelly B.

Director, Service Excellence

◇◇◇◇◇◇◇◇◇◇◇

"I have an open- and closed-door policy. Any time that I am here, I will make sure I have time for you if you need me. My closed-door policy is that we operate mutually respectfully in a public place. If you have something to say that is private, we come into my office, close the door and we have a discussion.

"Understand that the things that you get presented with are only one dimension of the issue. Don't react to the first thing you hear. Seek other points of view and reserve judgment."

Chris A.

Manager, Medical/Oncology

◇◇◇◇◇◇◇◇◇◇◇

"Protecting personal boundaries can be difficult in the manager role. In my experience, staff often forget that you have a life outside of the hospital. There have been times when the line has been crossed and it needs to be addressed immediately. In the management role, you are at the hospital and with the staff often more than you are with your own families. I believe it is the time spent and the relationships built that cause intrusion into personal boundaries.

"As a manager, you need to set the expectations and standards from the beginning. You need to truly make a list of what your expectations are and what you are willing to share with others. When those expectations are deviated from, then you need to have a candid conversation with the staff to let them know what behavior occurred and why it is not acceptable. I often find that open and honest communication has the best outcomes."

Tara M.

Manager, Adolescent Unit

◇◇◇◇◇◇◇◇◇◇

"I emphasize respect and utilizing the chain of command. I manage approximately 150 employees and continually make it known that we all have jobs, yet all have a life outside of work. I'm very supportive of staff, patients, physicians, and supervisors, but we all have a sense of respect for each other's time and time away from work. When I am at the hospital, my full attention is focused on meeting their needs, so I have learned to manage my time appropriately. It is a continual challenge every day though, due to patient leader rounding, hospital meetings, etc., etc., etc.!"

Morgan T.
Manager, PICC Team Clinical Unit

◇◇◇◇◇◇◇◇◇◇

"Do not friend any staff on social media! This is a great boundary for both you and your staff. I am always willing to listen to staff member's problems and offer resources that may help them. But at the end of every conversation, I bring the focus back to accountability for their role on the team and how are they going to meet the expectations of the role. We all have challenges and need support, but knowing what is expected and holding them accountable is the best way to grow a great nurse."

Tammy S.
Manager, Surgical Specialty Unit

◇◇◇◇◇◇◇◇◇◇

"The best piece of advice that I can give to other nurse managers for protecting their personal boundaries when dealing with the emotions and demands of staff, patients, physicians, and supervisors is to KNOW your personal boundaries. For me, in my practice, I feel it is very important to know what my boundaries are, and to what length they extend. My boundaries with a colleague of many years may be very different than my boundary with an employee that I have not known as long. Knowing oneself is so important when working with others, especially if we can only be responsible for our own responses to triggers."

Scott H.
Manager, Emergency Medicine & Trauma

◇◇◇◇◇◇◇◇◇◇

"I have struggled with boundaries. One thing that I found works is posting office hours that all I have planned is time with the staff. That is time for them. I find that if I have time alone for them, then they honor that and do not expect me here or to be available on my off-time. Assume good intent! When people come to you with an emotional issue, assume that they have good intent and that we can work on the process without emotion."

Desi S.
Manager, IMCU/PCU

◇◇◇◇◇◇◇◇◇◇

"Be objective and avoid subjective or judgmental statements. Try to identify the issue being represented by the behavior you're witnessing. People yell because they feel like they're not being heard. For example, if you have an employee who is upset about something and acting out, ask about what is causing their reaction and listen carefully to what they're both saying and not saying. Usually, if you start asking 'why' a few times, you'll start getting to the bottom of things.

"If the behavior is unprofessional (yelling, threatening, etc.), I specifically tell the person that I'm willing to work with them, but I will not tolerate being yelled at, and I will not tolerate my staff being yelled at (or threatened, or whatever the unacceptable behavior is). I then spend time listening to the person and hearing them out so they understand that yelling and acting out isn't necessary.

"There was a time when a doctor yelled at a nurse and called her a moron. I confronted the doctor by asking what occurred. He started off by yelling at me, which I immediately told him was unacceptable and informed him that I would listen to the problem so long as he stopped yelling. When he talked about the problem that he had, I acknowledged that he did hit a frustrating barrier, but that did not justify unprofessional behavior. When he asked what was unprofessional about his behavior, I informed him that I consider name-calling and raising voices on the patient care unit unprofessional and to refrain from doing so in the future.

"I then offered him an alternative by providing my contact information and instructions on how to properly escalate an issue when I'm not present in the hospital. I then made it clear that if such an event were to occur again, I would speak with the chair of his department, but that I expected this wouldn't be necessary now that we'd talked. I also acknowledged that I would promptly address any issues with my staff if they failed to meet the standard and that he should contact me if the issue occurred again."

Michelle K.
Manager of Emergency Community Operations

Your Thoughts?

Pick one or more of these examples of peer wisdom about boundaries to explore.
What lessons from your own experiences come to mind as you read these stories?

....

....

....

....

....

Q & Q: Quote and Question

Consider each quote about boundaries and answer the follow-up question from your experiences.

> Q: "Your personal boundaries protect the inner core of your identify and your right to choices."
>
> **Gerard Manley Hopkins**

Q: **How do your own personal boundaries influence your right to make choices in your leadership practice?**

....

....

....

....

> Q: "I have met the enemy and it is the eyes of other people."
>
> **Ben Franklin**

Q: **How do the imagined or real eyes of other people become the enemy of healthy boundaries?**

....

....

....

....

> Q: "No is a complete sentence."
>
> **Anne Lamott**

Q: **How is saying no connected to your creation of clear boundaries?**

....

....

....

....

> Q: "We need to re-create boundaries. When you carry a digital gadget that creates a virtual link to the office, you need to create a virtual boundary that didn't exist before."
>
> **Daniel Pink**

Q: **How do you create "virtual" boundaries with your cell phone, email, texting, Facebook page?**

....

....

....

....

> Q: "There is a huge amount of freedom that comes when you take nothing personally."
>
> **Tony Gaskin**

Q: **How would you interpret this statement in terms of your own experiences?**

....

....

....

....

> Q: "Do not let anyone walk through your mind with dirty feet."
>
> **Mahatma Gandhi**

Q: Can you think of a time when you let someone walk through your mind with dirty feet (e.g., bullying or shaming you), and a time when you stopped them?

....

....

....

....

 ## Deep Dive Resources: Boundaries

Books

Adams, J. (2005). *Boundary issues: Using boundary intelligence.* Wiley and Sons.

Black, J., & Enns, G. (1997). *Better boundaries: Owning and treasuring your life.* Raincoast Books.

Buchanan, G., & Seligman, M. (2009). *Explanatory styles.* Routledge.

Hartmann, E. (1991). *Boundaries in the mind: A new psychology of personality.* Basic Books.

Hochschild, A. R. (1997). *The time bind: When work becomes home and home becomes work.* Metropolitan Books.

Katherine, A. (2000). *Where to draw the line: How to set healthy boundaries every day.* Fireside.

Tawwab, N. (2021). *Set boundaries, find peace.* Penguin.

Professional Journals

Allen, D. (2000). The boundary work of a nurse manager in a district general hospital. *Journal of Contemporary Ethnography, 29*(3), 326–356.

Anderon, J., & Puckrin, K. (2011). Social network use: A test of self-regulation. *Journal of Nursing Regulation, 2*(1), 36-41.

Boswell, W. R., & Olson-Buchanan, J. B. (2007). The use of communication technologies after hours: The role of work attitudes and work-life conflict. *Journal of Management, 33*(4), 592–610.

Chreim, S., & Langley, A. (2013). Leadership boundary work in therapeutic teams. *Leadership, 9*(2), 201–228.

Holder, K. V., & Schenthal, S. J. (2007). Watch your step: Nursing and professional boundaries. *Nursing Management, 38*(2), 24–29.

Kreiner, G. E., Hollensbe, E. C., & Sheep, M. (2009). Balancing borders and bridges: Negotiating the work-home interface via boundary work tactics. *Academy of Management Journal, 52*(4), 704–730.

Klich-Heartt, E. I., & Prion, S. (2010). Social networking and HIPAA: Ethical concerns for nurses. *Nurse Leader, 8*(2), 56–58.

Sheets, V. R. (2000). Staying in the lines: Teach nurses how to maintain professional boundaries, recognize potential problems, and make better care decisions. *Nursing Management, 31*(8), 28–30.

Wright, L. D. (2006). Violating professional boundaries. *Nursing, 36*(3), 52–54.

Videos

Cloud, H. (2020, April 2). *How to set boundaries* [Video]. YouTube. https://www.youtube.com/watch?v=zjcPkKHZRCg

From the author of *Boundaries for Leaders.*

Tiedens, S. (2019, May 29). *Explanatory style* [Video]. YouTube. https://www.youtube.com/watch?v=JtNDcEqqj50

About Martin Seligman's Explanatory models.

Figure Credit

Fig. 3.1: Copyright © by Sally Deng. Reprinted with permission.

Self-Regulation

Master Emotional Overload

"To be a good manager and leader you really need to maintain your objectivity in very charged situations. One of the most important things that I have learned is to control my own affect when I'm angry or impatient. Because when you get emotional, you lose your objectivity. You say things that you regret; you don't do a good job."

◇◇◇◇◇◇◇◇◇◇◇◇◇◇◇◇

Rudyard Kipling's celebrated turn-of-the-century poem *If* may have been the first recorded job description of managing yourself: "If you can keep your head when all about you are losing theirs and blaming it on you ..."[1] Ninety years later, the godfathers of emotional intelligence, Peter Salovey, John Mayer, and Daniel Goleman, defined this capacity as self-regulation.[2,3] And it is also precisely what your colleague has described as "maintaining your objectivity" in charged situations.

Goleman describes self-regulation as an ongoing inner conversation, one that involves controlling or redirecting our disruptive emotions and impulses in order to make optimal decisions. He name-checks the behaviors: understanding your feelings—without being driven by them, suspending judgment, reflecting before acting, and staying focused on your priorities.

In other words, don't dance with anyone's amygdala. As Goleman explains, when two or more people are upset, each person's amygdala, the brain's stress driver, takes the wheel from the more rational, problem-solving prefrontal cortex. Heated interactions become a neural tug of war. The leader who takes command of his or her emotions, and conveys the sense that the situation can be managed, will win.

Kjung J. details the challenge: "Leaders are naturally passionate people; otherwise, we wouldn't pursue what is so dear to us. Yet keeping it cool is the number one criteria for being a successful leader. When we get excited, all the blood rushes out of our brains to our hearts and we can no longer think rationally. Introspection is an important asset when it comes to keeping it cool."

In this laboratory, we will explore three keys to meeting the challenges of self-regulation. These keys are grounded in the idea that self-regulation is both conscious and effortful—with behaviors that can be learned and practiced.[4,5] As you read, continue to reflect on your experiences and compare them with the ones that follow. Identify your best practices and plan to experiment with some new actionable strategies.

REFLECTION

What feelings does this painting evoke? What situations come to mind?

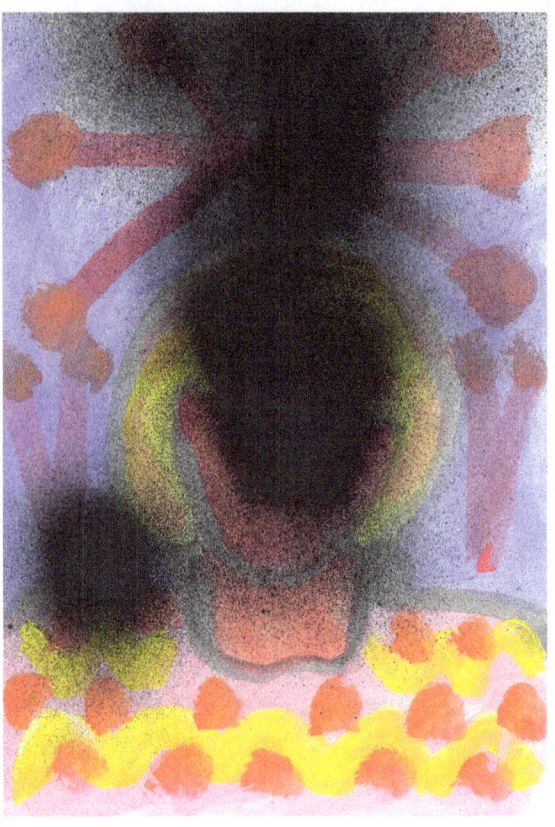

FIGURE 4.1

....

....

....

....

....

....

....

Three Keys to Meet the Challenge of Self-Regulation

Key	Strategies	Your best practices
Key #1 Rally your restraint.	~Stop the clock. ~Create imaginary distance. ~Rehearse an if/then plan. ~Plan to consult. ~Delegate to the committee of sleep.	
Key #2 Respond rather than react.	~Suspend judgment. ~Listen to understand. ~Conduct a self-scan. ~Consider your conclusions.	
Key #3 Reframe the situation.	~Employ positive explanatory models. ~Highlight core values. ~Assume positive intention. ~Review role model.	

REFLECTION

Describe a time with a team member, direct report, or patient when you met Kipling's criteria and "kept your head" when all around you were losing theirs. What were your strategies?

....

....

....

....

....

Next, describe an experience when you could not control your anger, anxiety, or impatience. What can you learn from the difference between the two outcomes?

....

....

....

....

....

What would you want to teach other leaders about what you learned?

....

....

....

....

....

Key #1: Rally Your Restraint

Whether dealing with snarky colleague or a team member who appears to be recovering from charisma bypass surgery, nurse leaders understand the value of the practice of restraint. "I have learned not to knee-jerk respond," said Stella G. For these leaders, it is the element of self-control that involves keeping emotions and impulses in check in order to clarify the situation and conserve energy for problem solving.

One manager admitted, "Sometimes it is learning when *not* to say something." And listen to Hallie K., who adopted the catchphrase of Helen Sinclair in Woody Allen's movie, *Bullets Over Broadway.* "When someone insults me, I have to tell myself: Do not speak."

Keeping your emotions in check involves a complex set of thoughts, words, and deeds. Among them is knowing when to withdraw and when to be silent, and how to keep your emotions in check in conversations when you feel angry, hurt, itchy, or threatened. This requires creating a demilitarized zone between charging into battle by overreacting and withdrawing from the field.

Organizational communication experts Kerry Patterson and Joseph Grenny have described two perilous ways to approach charged situations. Each response reduces the chances of participating in productive high-stakes conversations.[6] Many leaders, when they are emotionally aroused or attacked, will insist on their point of view by turning up the volume, overstating the case, bullying, or belittling the ideas of others.

Yet Patterson and Grenny also warn of the opposite reaction, that of complete withdrawal. If you choose to remain silent or mask your thoughts and feelings with sarcasm, you block the flow of mutual understanding needed to resolve the issue. Clearly, the key to restraint is a pause to refresh, followed by re-engagement.

But before you rally your restraint, explore what gets your goat. As the writer William Arthur Ward observed, "Whatever gets your goat gets your attention. Whatever gets your attention gets your time. Whatever gets your time gets you."

REFLECTION

Which situations or relationships are the biggest challenges to you in controlling strong feelings and "keeping your cool"? Which are the ones that take your time and attention? Jot down notes. Keep these in mind as you continue.

- A supervisor who is highly critical

....

....

....

....

....

- A provider who is rude or disrespectful toward you or a team member

....

....

....

....

....

- A colleague or direct report who is negative, divisive, or explosive

....

....

....

....

....

- A meeting that suddenly breaks bad

....

....

....

....

....

- A patient's family member who is angry, demanding, or complaining about your nursing or management team

....

....

....

....

....

- A challenge to your authority

....

....

....

....

....

REFLECTION

Consider an expression. Kristiina Junttilla, a Finnish nurse leader, taught me some kicky epressions for the American phrase "getting your goat." Finnish nurses, unable to control their strong feelings, would describe themselves as "burning my sleeves," "turning my cup upside down," or "putting a pea up my nose."[7]

What do these three expressions have in common? What is the message about self-regulation?

....

....

....

....

....

Your capacity to practice restraint, to avoid burning your sleeves, can depend on your willingness to take a pause that refreshes. This requires that you stop the clock. Referees and coaches understand the power of a short interruption in a game. They stop the clock so that the players may rest, deliberate, make substitutions, or halt a downward spiral. Begin by rejecting the idea that you must respond immediately to every situation.

"There is no problem in delaying an answer," counsels manager Randy W. "You have to be really willing to listen first, hear it all, think the whole picture through, and make a plan before you open your mouth. Because you will be sorry [if you react too quickly]."

The discussion of boundaries in Laboratory 3 touched on variations of "let me get back to you." You can press pause if you say, "Now, I have a clear sense of what your concerns are; give me some time to sort out what you have told me. Can you come by tomorrow morning?"

In the heat of the moment, experiment with a trio of slow-down strategies.

EXPERIMENT

Create an imaginary distance. Imagine sitting in the second balcony in a theater, looking down on your encounter. What would you see? Imagine the situation with the voiceover commentary of a sportscaster ("two strikes with bases loaded"), a weather reporter ("cloudy with a chance of meatballs"), or a red carpet host ("and *who* are you wearing?"). Adopt a mental hashtag (#Tryingnottoloseit), or imagine the conversation going viral on YouTube. Conjure your favorite comedian's take on the situation.

EXPERIMENT

Plan to consult. In the midst a heated encounter, pause and silently select a person with whom you can share the danger, the angst, and, yes, the humor of your current migraine moment.

Suzanne R. underlines this strategy. "We must have a safe place or safe individual where we can vent. Finding the peer or leader who becomes your sounding board to talk out your feelings and to review how you managed the situation is important. Sometimes we can't see plainly what needs to take place because we are too close to the situation."

You may best rally your restraint by delegating to the committee of sleep, advises psychologist William James, who reminds us that both restraint and creativity thrive on rest.[8] Sarah M. offers an example: "I recently had to speak with a travel RN, who was not known to be receptive to feedback, about her negative attitude and intense communication with me and her peers. Rather than speaking to her in the moment, I slept on it and spoke to her the following day."

"The next day, I intentionally kept my tone and body language relaxed and approached her from the point of view that I wanted to make sure we were still a good fit for her. We were then able to have an open conversation about her feeling overwhelmed. She acknowledged that she can become intense at times and that she wanted to work on this. I left the meeting feeling good about pushing through apprehensive feelings and doing something that was difficult."

Remember that self-possession in sweaty moments takes practice. Psychologist Peter Gollwitzer, who has studied the gap between our intentions and our actual behavior, suggests a mental rehearsal approach he describes as "if-then."[9]

The application here is that, when you know are going into a potential sticky situation, you can create and rehearse a series of if-then statements.

Imagine that you have scheduled a meeting with a colleague who groans at your every suggestion. You intention is to let him know how this affects you, your expectation for him to behave in a more collaborative way, and how this will enhance your relationship. When you have carefully planned what you will say, you would also plan what to do and say *if* you go off script, getting shouty, taking the bait or upping the ante.

REFLECTION

Describe a troubling situation or stressful conversation on your horizon.

. . . .

. . . .

. . . .

. . . .

. . . .

Write an if-then plan that allows you to rehearse an outcome—in case your behavior creates a detour from your original intention.

. . . .

. . . .

. . . .

. . . .

. . . .

Key #2: Respond Rather Than React

Suspending judgment and thinking before acting are crucial to self-regulation. Managers often label this as an act of patience—one they accomplish through their deliberate slowing-down of their reaction times and in-depth listening. "You need to take it all in, before you react to situations," said one leader. "I think listening is a form of patience," said another. "It is a way of buying time so that you are not reacting. If it is a nurse, I will say, 'Tell me more about what happened.' If it is a patient or family member, I just listen to what they have to say."

Donna G. drills down the specifics. "It often means listening differently, asking questions, not arriving at a judgment without enough information. But really being open to that particular human being and their take on it, even though I'm thinking, 'Gee whiz, what happened? How did we get there?' Then I have to make sure that I get it and understand what they were doing, so that's part of the patience; to take a deep breath and say, 'Tell me more, I don't quite understand.'"

Slowing down allows for the process of metacognition—you can think about your thoughts. Psychologists Aaron Beck and David Burns, who study how distorted thought patterns drive outcomes, urge us to recognize what they call "automatic negative thoughts" that can make a bad situation worse.[10, 11] Among them are all-or-nothing thinking, over generalization, speedy conclusions, disqualifying the positive, self-blame, and shame.

EXPERIMENT

Suspend judgment by listening to understand. Mitchell Rabkin, the former CEO of Beth Israel Hospital in Boston, calls this "getting the whole story." He describes the stakes: "Once you voice an opinion, you can't get too emotionally attached to it in the face of the facts. If you are not willing to take in another point of view and change yours, you are in deep yogurt."[12] Rabkin's counsel suggests that you listen before you reply, by asking, "What do I need to know to understand?" and "How do *you* see this situation?"

REFLECTION

Recall a time when you reacted at the speed of light and acted upon a judgment without having enough information. Did you engage in any automatic negative thought patterns? Were you too attached to your point of view and unable to take another perspective?

....

....

....

....

....

Rewrite the story of that situation and give it a different ending. What questions could you have asked that would have contributed to a more positive outcome?

....

....

....

....

....

EXPERIMENT

Conduct a self-scan. Leadership educator Adele Lynn has outlined a four-point check-list to raise self-awareness during times of emotional overload.[13] Focus on the physical: Do you have a clenched jaw, dry mouth, sweaty hands, or racing heartbeat? Next, quickly acknowledge your feelings: Are you anxious? Angry? Defensive? Scared? Impatient? Now, imagine how you might appear to others: Exasperated? Disappointed? Withdrawn? Nurse Jackie on steroids? Last, scan your thoughts. Are you defending your position or discrediting others? How might you be distorting the situation with one of the automatic negative thought patterns Burns describes?

EXPERIMENT

Consider your conclusions. Communications expert Judith Glaser takes the self-scan one step further, and outlines a way to study your steps on the ladder to mistaken and messy conclusions.[14] Let's envision a dust-up with the on-call resident—the one who questioned your decision about a patient.

Glaser suggests that you begin the jump to conclusions by noting your bio-reaction. ("My heart is hammering.") You then label the interaction in terms of how bad or good you feel. ("I feel humiliated.") Next, you put words to your feelings and make up a story to assign meaning to the situation. ("I have been here all day, and he wants to barge in and tell me what to do.") Finally, you pull in other beliefs to underline your conclusion. ("He is just like most residents; he has no respect for what nurses do.") With this conclusion, driven only by feelings, there is little chance that you can take command of the situation.

REFLECTION

Return to the situation you described above—one where you jumped to conclusions. Begin a fact check. You might ask, What evoked my intense reaction? What assumptions was I making? Were my assumptions beliefs or facts? Was my strong reaction proportionate to the facts of the situation? Or was I giving a $500 reaction a $50 stimulus? If so, why?

....

....

....

....

....

Key #3: Reframe the Situation

Anger, anxiety, and negativity are contagious. The practice of self-management requires that your feelings about situations be understood and framed in a way that allows you to master them. As Dana R. explains, "If you stay with negativity and complaints, then your hair will always be exploding. If you walk about like that, your staff turns into that. If they see your hair is on fire, their hair is on fire too."

A Chinese proverb puts this another way: You cannot keep the bird of sorrow from flying over your head, but you can prevent it from making a nest in your hair.

Psychologist Robert Kegan explains that reframing takes place in the zone between the actual event (the sad bird flying overhead) and our reaction to it (whether it makes a home in our hair).[15] Martin Seligman and Glen Elder's groundbreaking research on optimistic and pessimistic explanatory models offers the blueprint by comparing two ways of explaining, framing, and mastering emotionally demanding experiences.[16] The shiny idea here is that self-regulation is driven by your inner dialogue about the situation and how you describe the situation to yourself and others.

Imagine this: A member of your team, and someone who you have prized and nurtured, has quit unexpectedly. A pessimistic framework would see the situation as *permanent* ("We can never get this project done without her."), *pervasive* ("We're doomed. This is going to ruin everything ..."), and *personal* ("How could she do this to me? I thought I was her mentor. It's all my fault! If had paid more attention, I would have seen this coming.").

In Seligman and Elder's perspective, an optimistic framework would describe the situation in a way that conveys mastery and the belief that the challenge can be met. They describe three hallmarks of optimistic thought: language that describes the problem as *temporary* ("It will be rough for a few weeks until we replace her."), *specific* ("She was working on new nurse orientation. Who can cover there until we hire someone?"), and *objective* ("Many people leave jobs, even when they have had lots of support. But in the future, I think I'll do more climate checks.").

 REFLECTION

Select a recent challenge or charged encounter—one that raised your blood pressure.

....

....

....

....

....

First, explain it with a pessimistic framework (permanent-pervasive-personal).

Permanent:

....

....

....

....

....

Pervasive:

....

....

....

....

Personal:

....

....

....

Next, explain it with an optimistic framework (temporary-specific-objective).

Temporary:

....

....

....

....

....

Specific:

....

....

....

....

Objective:

....

....

....

....

Describe your observation about each of the two explanations.

....

....

....

....

....

EXPERIMENT

Positive explanatory models are also a powerful silent framework that allow you to choose your thoughts—and drive the actions that result from them. So do not believe everything you think, and work to change your conversation with yourself.

Instead of thinking, "I will never be able to approach them," try, "This will take planning and effort." Rather than silently fuming, "He is just jealous because he wanted my job," you might wonder, "How can I work with him—knowing he is disappointed that I got the job he wanted?"

Kelly G. a prefers a shorthand framework she calls "Q-Tip." Translation: "Quit taking it personally."

EXPERIMENT

Reframe by highlighting your values and intentions rather than your feelings. Clinical psychologist Steven Stosny has observed that self-regulation is more attainable when it emphasizes values rather than feelings.[17] When we center attention on our feelings, this focus amplifies, magnifies, and distorts them. In this light, self-regulation is the ability to act in your long-term best interest, consistent with your deepest values.

Todd G. poses a wise question. "I ask myself: Is this about my values or kindness? If not, it's likely about ego and feeling like someone isn't 'respecting you or your department.' So I let it go."

In a stormy get-together with two angry nurses, Miranda H. reframed and maintained her composure by focusing on her core concerns. "I gathered all the information and focused on three things: What is best for the patients we were caring for? What is best for each of these staff members? And how do we resolve this issue and prevent future occurrences?"

EXPERIMENT

Discover a theory of relativity. If Einstein's goal was to convince his fellow physicists that there were no absolutes in the universe, your goal is to manage to put challenging events and personalities in a relative perspective.

Here are two examples from your colleagues: "When I get impatient, I try to remember the only time anything around here happens quickly is when there is a code. And there is no *management* code," joked Brenda R. Todd G. creates perspective by "thinking, what will this mean to me next week? I keep repeating in my head over and over: It's no big deal. ... It's no big deal."

Theories of relativity allow you to avoid battle fatigue. As Sharon B. puts it, "I learned to choose my battles and not to choose losing battles. If you know you are going to lose the battle, don't waste your time fighting it. Sometimes I had to give up things that I thought I wanted for the greater good—to turn the situation into something that is good for the hospital, for me and for my team."

 REFLECTION

What might happen if you lowered the temperature of an encounter by considering and suggesting a generous interpretation of a team member's behavior? For Kate M., assuming positive intention is a powerful habit of mind in her leadership.[18] "I treat people like they had the best of intentions, even if they didn't. And that's just how I think. But I do it intentionally, too. If somebody does something—and it seems counterproductive to the team—I will see it as, 'You were trying to help that patient, weren't you?' I give them a way to say it, to show that they had good intentions."

How might this idea influence your leadership practice?

....

....

....

....

....

We close with two less poetic "ifs" than Rudyard Kipling's. What if you counted to 100, reframed with optimism, suspended judgment, hewed to your values, and you still sent the raging email or let the dogs out? What if your staff member, despite your coaching, unloads her frustration on a patient's less-than-charming daughter? In these situations, Suzanne R. observes, "We can either choose to beat ourselves up for not handling a situation well or learn from the experience and move forward."

Marle S. reminds us that all of our failures at self-regulation are opportunities to leverage lessons. She redefines what it means for both you and your staff to keep "a cool head." It means keeping your eye on the goal, understanding that there will be bumps along the way, and taking advantage of learning from those bumps.

She describes the drill. "When interacting with your team members, try to remember that we are *all* works in progress. They *will* disappoint you. Keep your cool and keep mentoring. Nothing is more rewarding than seeing team member learn from their mistakes and grow as a nurse, as an employee, and as a human being."

Marle's inspiration for self-regulation is to remember your best role models. "At some point in your career, you have probably disappointed a leader. Did your leader *lose their cool* with you? What did they do to help you learn all you could from that situation, and ensure that the next time around, you made a better decision?"

Her advice about emotional mastery invites us to be well-measured and wise.

Ask a Nurse Leader: Peer Wise Ideas About Self-Regulation

Pick one or more of these examples of peer wisdom about self-regulation to explore. What lessons from your own experience come to mind as you read these stories?

◇◇◇◇◇◇◇◇◇◇

"What has worked for me is spending 15 minutes each day after I go home from work to think about my day and how I feel about it. I try to figure out whether I'm satisfied or rather frustrated about how the day went and the reason for how I'm feeling. Once I figure out why I'm feeling the way I'm feeling, I can figure out what my next step is.

"Self-control is not always easy. I also spend the first few minutes of each morning reading a code of leadership. My covenant changes depending on what I feel I need to work on. These are my recent reminders of leadership to myself:

"Talk less, listen more. Be inclusive, by getting others' input. I don't have to prove I know all the answers or am smarter than others. Seek to understand so that I may be understood. Be kind. Be patient.

"Leadership is a constant battle—with myself, always striving to be a better person than I was yesterday. I also try to be kind and forgiving of me, since I can be my worst enemy. I have been a manager for 9 years now and I am a better person. I hope I am a better manager."

Kyung J.
OR Manager

◇◇◇◇◇◇◇◇◇◇

"In today's fast-paced and excellence-driven health care environment, nurse managers have demanding jobs. Stressful situations can occur on an almost daily basis. Knowing the stressful health care environment in which we exist today, I often ask new job applicants to tell me of a time they have been involved in conflict. 'Tell me a little about the situation and how you handled it.' When I hear the answer 'I don't have conflict,' I know they are not being honest. We all deal with conflict in our jobs and we have two options, either chose to ignore or take some type of action.

"When I am faced with an emotionally charged and stressful situation, I try to hear the other party out before making a judgment. Is the person acting out because they are stressed themselves? Do they need to be validated or have they been wronged? Understanding what is going on many times helps to de-escalate the situation and also helps me not make preconceived assumptions of the other person. On the other hand, if this situation is taking place in a staff meeting and is not beneficial to the group, I ask the individual to see me after the meeting to discuss further. If the situation is taking place within hearing of a patient or their family, I pull them aside privately and have the discussion above.

"If the emotionally charged situation is directed toward me, individually, I hear the other person out and acknowledge if they have been wronged. If needed in the situation, I take the time to point out the need to remain professional in our communication. I make sure to let them know how the conversation made me feel instead of using 'you' blaming. I then turn the situation around and ask them how they would feel if it happened to them or one of their loved ones in that manner. I reflect upon our organizational values of treating each other with dignity and respect in all situations.

"Furthermore, we must have a 'safe place or safe individual' that we can vent to. Finding that peer or leader that becomes your sounding board to talk out your feelings and to review with you how you managed the situation is important. Sometimes we can't see plainly what needs to take place because we are too close to the situation. I am glad I have this individual in my professional life!

"Another way to destress is to take a walk or run, or to participate in some type of physical activity several times a week, especially after a stressful day. It is also a good way to reflect upon what happened during the day and let it go. … Each day is a new learning opportunity for growth. We can either choose to beat ourselves up for not handling a situation well or learn from the experience and move forward."

Suzanne R.
Manager, Trauma Unit

◇◇◇◇◇◇◇◇◇◇◇

"In my experience as a leader, learning to keep a cool head in our challenging environments is something that requires practice. Being a good leader is *frustrating* at times. One of my mentors told me on my first day as a manager, 'Marle, prepare for daily disappointment!' And she was right.

"Disappointment can often lead to anger and resentment. Leading means having a vision of realizing the *potential* of your department and staff. But people are people. They will make bad decisions, they will choose the easier way at times, they will disappoint you. However, if that were the end of the story, none of us would stick it out. If 'daily disappointment' is part of the job, *WHY* do we keep showing up every day? Because, although staff, providers, and even other leaders disappoint you, as a LEADER **YOU** have the power to coach and mentor that person into making a better decision the next time.

"You also have the privilege to recognize people within your organization for doing the RIGHT thing, for taking the tougher route, and for taking a stand. Some of my most fulfilling times as a leader have been to watch low or struggling performers learn and grow under good mentorship. To blow up and lose my cool when those staff members disappointed me may have prevented learning from occurring, or damaged, forever, the relationship and trust I had built with that person.

"So although my mentor did share with me that disappointment would be my constant companion as a leader, she failed to mention that *successes*, both little and groundbreaking, would also be a daily occurrence. Keeping a cool head means keeping your eye on the goal, understanding that there will be bumps along the way, and taking advantage of learning from those *bumps*. When interacting with your staff members, try to remember that we are ALL works in progress. They *will* disappoint you. Keep your cool and keep mentoring. Nothing is more rewarding than seeing a staff member learn from their mistakes and grow as a nurse, as an employee, and as a human being. Keeping a cool head can turn a conversation you have with an employee from a frustrating, disappointing experience to a rewarding learning opportunity between you and your staff member."

Marle S.
Manager, Labor & Delivery

◇◇◇◇◇◇◇◇◇◇◇

"One of my female role models is Eleanor Roosevelt. Three of my favorite quotes that guide me through tough situations: 'No one can make you feel inferior without your consent.' 'A woman is like a tea bag—you can't tell how strong she is until you put her in hot water.' 'You gain strength, courage, and confidence by every experience in which you really stop to look fear in the face.'

"I have been in management for 18 years. And through the years, I have learned to face challenges as lessons to be learned. Someone is trying to teach me something about myself. [It is a] lesson in introspection. No matter the chaos or the behaviors displayed for me to witness, I challenge myself by assessing whether I have the skills to bring the individual or the environment back to equilibrium.

"As the lesson unfolds in front of me, I listen carefully to the 'presenter' (the individual who has a grievance). I ask questions for clarity and understanding of the material being presented. By doing such, the individual usually calms down. We talk over the issues and we leave with an agreement for a current or future state."

Thu J.
Assistant Director

◇◇◇◇◇◇◇◇◇◇◇

"I think this question is two-fold. I'm a big proponent of work–life balance. There is nothing wrong with thinking about yourself and ensuring you are in the best place mentally and physically. I have the opportunity to have unit managers 'report' (I don't like that word because I think it's more collaboration) to me and there have been times where I have had to mandate them to go home. Not because they were doing a poor job, but they needed to take time for themselves and regroup—there's nothing wrong with that. Though in nursing I think we could do a way better job of work–life balance in general!

Second is to always maintain professionalism and don't take offense. Above all else, you are a leader and your staff sees you as a role model. There will be times when co-workers or other departments will get under your skin and you might take offense. Many times it's because these departments or co-workers don't understand nursing's role or process. It's our job to explain nursing's role in the organization to other departments and how our work affects patients."

Gretchen P.
Director of Surgical and Multispecialty Services

Your Thoughts?

Pick one or more of these examples of peer wisdom about self-regulation to explore. What lessons from your own experiences come to mind as you read these stories?

....

....

....

....

....

Q & Q: Quote and Question

Consider each quote about self-regulation and self-control and answer the follow-up question from your own experiences.

> Q: "I will be calm. I will be mistress of myself."
>
> **Jane Austen, *Sense and Sensibility***

Q: Can you describe a time in your practice when self-regulation allowed you to be the mistress/master of yourself? What are the thoughts and behaviors that allowed you to remain calm?

....

....

....

....

> Q: "If you are distressed by anything external, the pain is not due to the thing itself, but to your estimate of it; and this you have the power to revoke at any moment."
>
> **Marcus Aurelius**

Q: Evaluate the value of this statement from the perspective of your own experience. Can you think of a time when your estimate of the situation—the way you explained it to yourself—increased or lessened the pain of the situation?

....

....

....

....

Q: "Speak when you are angry and you will make the best speech you will ever regret."

Ambrose Bierce

Q: Can you describe a situation in your experience that illustrates this idea, where you spoke out of anger? Can you rewrite the situation and give it a different ending?

....

....

....

....

Q: "I think one's feelings waste themselves in words; they ought all to be distilled into actions which bring results."

Florence Nightingale

Q: Can you think of a time when you translated your feelings (frustration, anger, grief, joy) into an actionable strategy—one that brought positive results?

....

....

....

....

> Q: "It is a common experience that a problem difficult at night is resolved in the morning after the committee of sleep has worked on it."
>
> **John Steinbeck**

Q: Describe a situation that you "slept on" that was easier to resolve the next day.

....

....

....

....

 ## Deep Dive Resources: The Practice of Self-Regulation

Books

Bradberry, T., & Greaves, J. (2009). *Emotional intelligence 2.0.* Talent Smart.

Cherniss, C., & Goleman. D. (Eds.). (2001). *The emotionally intelligent workplace: How to select for, measure, and improve emotional intelligence in individuals, groups, and organizations.* Jossey-Bass.

Codier, E. (2020). *Emotional intelligence in nursing: Essentials for leadership and practice improvement.* Springer.

Glaser, K. (2014). *Conversational intelligence.* Bibliomotion.

Goleman, D. (2006). *Working with emotional intelligence.* Bantam Books.

Lynn, A. (2002). *The emotional intelligence activity book: 50 activities for promoting eq at work.* HRD Press.

Moss, M. (2005). *The emotionally intelligent nurse leader.* Jossey Bass.

Patterson, K., Grenny, J., McMillan, R., & Switzler, A. (2012). *Crucial conversations: Tools for talking when the stakes are high.* McGraw Hill.

Professional Journals

Akerjordet, K., & Severinsson, E. (2008). Emotionally intelligent nurse leadership: A literature review study. *Journal of Nursing Management, 16*(5), 56–57.

Amendolair, D. (2003). Emotional intelligence: Essential for developing nurse leaders. *Nurse Leader, 1*(6), 25–27.

Bulmer-Smith, B., Profetto-McGrath, J., & Cummings, G. G. (2009). Emotional intelligence and nursing: An integrative literature review. *International Journal of Nursing Studies, 46*(12), 1625–1635.

Codier, E. E., Muneno, L., Franey, K., & Matsuura, F. (2010). Is emotional intelligence an important concept for nursing practice? *Journal of Psychiatric and Mental Health Nursing, 17*(10), 940–948.

Coladonato, A. (2017). Nurse leader emotional intelligence: How does it affect clinical nurse job satisfaction? *Nursing Management, 48*(9), 2–33.

Kooker, M. B., Shoultz, J., & Codier, E. (2007). Identifying emotional intelligence in professional nursing practice. *Journal of Professional Nursing, 23*(1), 30–36.

Mularz, L. A., & Johansen, M. L. (2016). An educational program to promote emotional mastery skills in nurse managers. *Journal for Nurses in Professional Development, 32*(3), E1–E7.

Vitello-Cicciu, J. M. (2003). Innovative leadership through emotional intelligence. *Nurse Manager, 34*(10), 29–32.

Video and Audio

Callibrain. (2015, August 20). Video review for crucial conversations by Kerry Patterson [Video]. YouTube. https://www.youtube.com/watch?v=EFaXx3pgaxM

Wolfe, C. (Host). (2013, January 30). Center for Emotional Intelligence at Yale University [Audio story]. PRX. https://beta.prx.org/stories/91799?play=true

Emotional Road Map with Mark Bracket, PhD, Director of the Center for Emotional Intelligence at Yale University.

Figure Credit

Generativity

Nurture the Next Generation

"I love the aha moments, when everything falls into place for the new nurse—when you are getting ready for their first-year evaluation and you see them with a smile on their face and their attitude is: 'I've got this, I can do this. I didn't make the biggest mistake in my life!'

"They look at ease as they are leaving from night shift or arriving on dayshift. They are at peace with being a nurse. This keeps me working for them, and the new ones to come. Most jobs are just jobs; this job changes lives while saving them."

◇◇◇◇◇◇◇◇◇◇◇◇◇◇◇

Your colleague has gifted us with an exuberant story of her practice of *generativity*—defined by psychoanalyst Erick Erickson as the concern for establishing and guiding the next generation.[1] Her joy in nurturing autonomy and identifying with the success of her team demonstrates generative concern as well as generative behavior.[2] In this laboratory, we will explore both the attitude and strategies for the practice of generativity in your leadership.

First a little background: In his landmark studies of the stages of adult development and identity in the 1950s, Erik Erikson used the word generativity to describe what he saw as a life stage that was a milestone of maturity—one where adults were ready to look beyond their own lives and invest in the next generation. He concluded that this milestone was a crucible of contentment in late adulthood; it was preventative medicine to avoid stagnation and self-absorption.

In the decades that followed, social scientists embraced the notion of generativity but agreed to disagree with Erikson's idea that its practitioners were all members of AARP. For example, psychologist John Kotre's work on legacy widened the definition to include our desire to invest in forms of life and work that will outlive us.[3] Most notably, the elegant and moving research of Edward de St. Aubin and Dan McAdams yielded dimensions of generative behavior and a persuasive argument that it could be expressed throughout adult life.[4, 5]

Drawing from a database of subjects who worked at an urban hospital, a university, a supermarket, and a social agency, they identified several intentions in action that create the practice of generativity. Among them are creating a legacy in one's image, cultivating and preserving ideas that link generations, offering up what has been created and maintained to the next generation as a gift, and finally, liberating this gift with its own autonomy and freedom.

De St. Aubin and McAdams also seconded the emotions of your colleague, suggesting that those who give the gift of generativity will receive many happy returns.

REFLECTION

Describe a nurse leader in your past—someone who guided you with generative concern and behavior. Note how they passed on the wisdom of their experience.

....

....

....

....

....

How did they embolden you to discover your strengths and meet your challenges?

....

....

....

....

....

How did they convey pride and praise about your work?

....

....

....

....

....

Name the ways they offered you new opportunities and autonomy, and honored your choices.

....

....

....

....

....

Generativity and Mentorship

So how is the practice of generativity different from mentoring? The extensive literature of mentoring describes intentional, supportive, one-to-one connections.[6, 7] Generativity, in contrast, is a more global set of attitudes and actions aimed at guiding multiple members of younger generations.

The vocabulary of pratice defines several braided features. *Generative concern* is described as the overall orientation or attitude regarding the wish to invest in, and care for, the next generation. *Generative commitment* is evidenced by decision making and goal setting that seeks to take responsibility for the next generation. *Generative action* refers to specific behaviors that promote the well-being of future generations.[8]

Clearly, mentoring is one specific expression of these three facets. Researchers Andrea McCloughen Louise O'Brien and Debra Jackson have captured the marriage of mentorshop and generativity in their evocative descriptions of the nurse leader mentor experience as "a mode of being."[9] They link the word *mode* to its Latin roots of *modus*: measure, extent, quantity, rhythm, a way, manner, fashion, style.

Four Keys to Generative Behavior

Keep your lived experiences of your own generativity in mind—its rhythm, music, and measures—as you examine four keys to generative behavior. Identify your best practices and plan to experiment with actionable strategies to enrich your leadership.

Key	Strategies	Your best practices
Key #1 Invest in their success.	~Learn to identify with the growth of your team. ~Recognize the losses of leadership. ~Consider what you create.	
Key #2 Create a legacy of care.	~Tell them a story. ~Become a teacher of meaning. ~Work out loud.	
Key #3 Engage in acts of random guidance.	~Hold up the mirror. ~Be particular in your praise. ~Ask; don't just tell.	
Key #4 Embolden with opportunity and autonomy.	~Explore your resistance. ~Provoke leadership. ~Encourage the yet.	

Key #1: Invest in Their Success

Kara T. bought a sponge in the hospital gift shop—the kind that grows to 10 times its size. "When this gets big enough to take over my job, I'm done. I am growing a boss," she said. Kara's capacity to find satisfaction and enjoyment in watching others develop is the driving force of generativity.

Kara's sponge is a kicky example of what Erickson described as choosing creative investment in others over stagnation and self-absorption. Leaders confirm the emotional income of their vested interest. "It is watching people grow and knowing that you are a part of that," said one leader. Another explained, "Our nurses are just so bright and they go from being a new grad to running a committee by themselves or going to great lengths to make something different for a patient. To see that growth is one of the best parts of the job."

Clearly, the generativity of these leaders is powered by identification—the capacity to locate your success as a leader in the accomplishments of others.[10] For some of us, the satisfaction is spontaneous; for others, it must be cultivated and practiced.

Consider the challenge. Because much of your work is accomplished through others, you may experience a significant sense of loss. As you move into various levels of leadership, the satisfactions of your devotion to bedside patient care have been replaced with tasks and goals of leadership. Cindy L. explains the shift. "If something happens and one of my nurses gets the credit, I just sit back and enjoy that."

For this reason, the practice of generativity—grounded in your identification with the attainments of your teams at the bedside—is a key to your ongoing engagement as a leader. David H. describes this attitude adjustment: "I used to think that I should really go back to bedside nursing—where you can affect your assignment of patients for a day. But now as a manager, I affect 52 staff people. To me, the influence in terms of giving [allows me to have much more of an input]."

There is more. Identification enables you to reinvigorate your standards of success by including a view of your achievements in light of the triumphs of your team. As Veda S. explains, "I feel that I am accomplishing things when I can see a team member grow, become more confident, and want to do new things. When I see someone take pride in what they do and hear others praise them, that keeps me excited about my role as a nurse leader."

 REFLECTION

Study Bhari Longs's painting, *Passing on the Baton*. What is gained and lost when you pass on power and knowledge to members of your team?

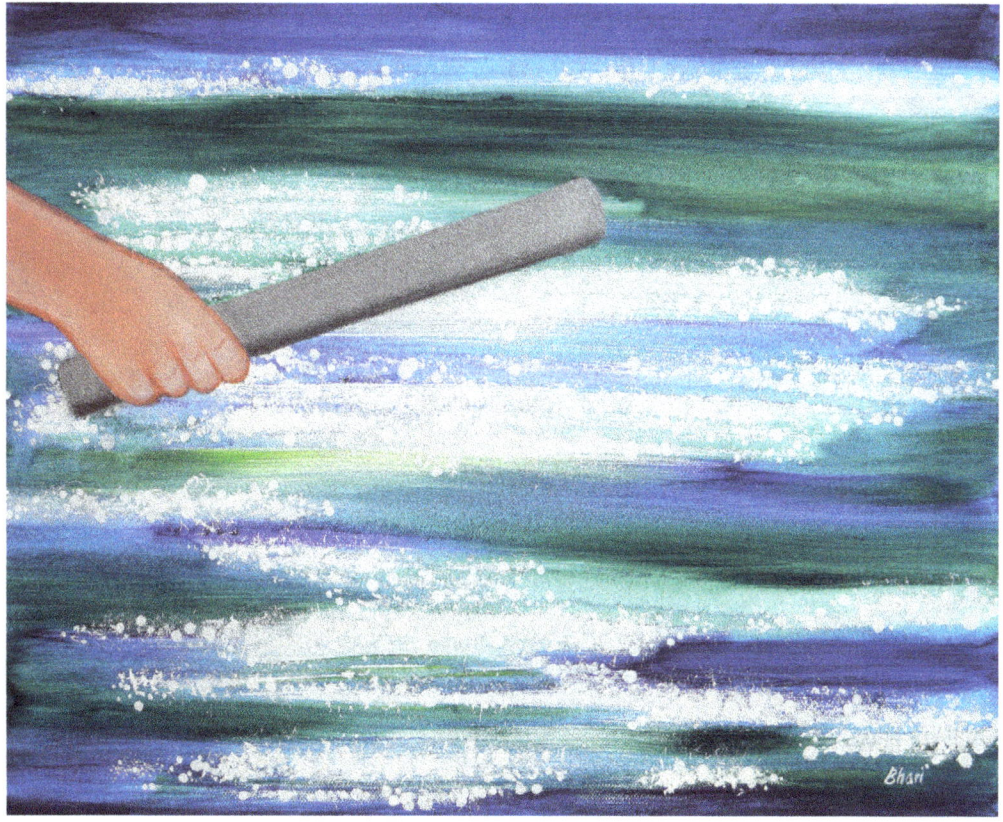

FIGURE 5.1

....

....

....

REFLECTION

Listen to a story from Joan D.: "I find that the most rewarding time is when you see someone whom you have been mentoring into a lead position suddenly does not need to ask any questions regarding their role as a leader. When they come to my office, it's not to ask how to do anything, but just to visit and let me know how things are."

First consider: What are the reasons for Joan's sense of pride? What has Joan gained?

....

....

....

....

What has she lost by declaring a team member's independence?

....

....

....

....

How is this an example of mutual motivation?

....

....

....

....

EXPERIMENT

Behold what you create. Henry David Thoreau wrote, "It is something to be able to paint a ... picture, or to carve a statue, ... so to make a few objects beautiful; but it is far more glorious to carve and paint the very atmosphere ... through which we [work] ... [t]o affect the quality of the day."[11]

Each week, take note of all of the ways that you "carve and paint" an environment that allows your team to contribute to a healing environment for patients and their families.

Key #2: Create a Legacy of Care

The Japanese language uses the evocative phrase *sedai-keisho-sei* to speak about generativity. *Sedai* means the "generations," *keisho* means "receiving and expressing in your own way," and *sei* can be translated as "the sense of."[12] To wit: When you express generativity, you receive something from the past, you create something from what you have learned, and you pass it on to the future.

Nurse leaders underline this process of passing on what they have received and understood from the past. Two pithy examples: "I see myself imprinted on them, almost like a mother duck." "I really like getting the new ones in here and getting them started and giving them the enthusiasm that I have." These two leaders—who shared the wisdom of their experiences with a younger generation—have created an extension of themselves and their standards of practice that will outlive their own presence on the job.

In his research about legacy, John Kotre described technical knowledge (passing on specific skills) and cultural wisdom (passing on lessons of values and meaning).[13] Melanie K.'s sense of legacy includes both: "I was able to stay in a leadership role because I thought of the position as a way of making sure the people were taken care of the way I'd want them to be taken care of."

Kotre has also written with refreshing candor about the incremental growth of generativist practice in the life of iconic nurse Florence Nightingale. He described the Nightingale School and Home for Nurses in London, where aspiring nurses were evaluated with both a moral and a technical report card.

He points out that in her seminal book, *Notes on Nursing,* Nightingale alternated between passing on technical details and standards ("Never let a patient be waked out of his first sleep") and cultural canons of nursing ("A nurse must be a sound, close and quick observer ... a woman of delicate and decent feeling").[14]

Stacy L., who manages a pediatric unit, has made the generative transition from being a holder of meaning to become a teacher of culture and meaning. "I'll tell [my staff] the kids come first and it begins with each of us. And I have service principles that I share. Some of it is basic, being polite, and some of it is extending yourself and putting yourself in the shoes of these families, or the children, or your employees, so that you can work with them to achieve their goals."

REFLECTION

Consider your leadership practice in terms of a legacy for future generations. Explore the meaning of *sedai-keisho-sei* in your own development.

Describe the most important technical (skills) and cultural lessons (values and meaning) that you have received in your years of practice.

....

....

....

....

....

How have you, or could you, translate these lessons (in your own terms) and pass them on to your team?

....

....

....

....

....

REFLECTION

Compare notes with Zoe H., who describes the satisfactions of working with "the first nurse I interviewed, I chose, I hired, and mentored." She elaborates, "I realized the fact that I was actually shaping her future. She was just starting out on her first job. She had no preconceived notion; she didn't know what to expect. I helped guide her and helped show her what nursing was really like here at this hospital, as well as in the community."

Describe the first nurse you brought into the embrace of your legacy as a nurse leader. What did you want to teach them? How did that early experience inform and shape your future leadership?

....

....

....

....

....

EXPERIMENT

Tell them a story. Your stories can be leveraged to demonstrate learning from experience (see Laboratory #1) as well as a way of modeling and passing on your values.[15]

CNO Jeannette E. told the story of being a novice nurse and being ridiculed by a surgeon for a mistake in her wound care. Not only did she describe the experience, she also expressed how she made sense of that situation. "I never forgot the feeling of humiliation. And I was determined that I would never make anyone feel that way."

REFLECTION

Return to your reflections in Laboratory #1. Is there a meaningful story you have—or could have—told your team as a way of passing on the wisdom of your experience?

....

....

....

....

....

Work out loud. Generative leaders must be seen and heard. Darla M. still remembers: "My very first supervisor taught me everything I could know about nursing—in the way she performed things. She would say, 'This is how you make people feel better: Instead of giving them a sedative, you do peri-care before they go to bed.' She went in and did the care, even though she was a supervisor. Nothing was a small task for her; she taught me that small things make a difference."[16]

Key #3: Engage in Random Acts of Guidance

Nurse leader Debra Jackson suggests that generativity can be expressed in acts of professional generosity.[17] She calls these "random acts of guidance" because they do not need to be framed or contained in a formal mentor relationship. She is bullish on the value and significance of a solitary nurturing or guiding act in a single encounter.

REFLECTION

Describe a time when a supervisor, preceptor, or teacher nurtured your development with a random act of guidance.

....

....

....

....

....

Hold up the mirror. Your team members see themselves reflected in your eyes. When you see something, say something. Show them that you see the unique strengths they bring. As Greg E. explained, "Often, people have a very limited view of themselves, and they need us, like a mirror, to show them qualities they are yet to appreciate."

EXPERIMENT

Be particular in your praise. Laboratory #2 explored the motivating potential of specific praise. Express generative guidance by using specific adjectives to describe the strengths of a member of your team. Match each of these ten words with someone on your team and seek the opportunity to tell them the qualities that you see.

- Accepting: meets people where they are; accepts many viewpoints
- Articulate: expresses thoughts and feelings clearly
- Flexible: rolls with the punches
- Insightful: can shed light on the heart of an issue or relationship
- Good humored: helps us see the lighter side
- Open minded: receptive to new ideas, diverse views
- Resourceful: knows where to look when ideas or tools are needed
- Persistent: perseveres in spite of obstacles
- Empathic: listens to understand, rather than just respond
- Passionate: devoted to mission and values of organization—to the patients you serve

EXPERIMENT

Create "ask, don't just tell" performance evaluations. Once you have covered the metrics your organization requires, you can pose enriching guiding questions. Send one or more of these questions in advance via email and explore them in a generous, nurturing discussion.

- How does your work contribute to our success?
- What is it like to work on this team?
- What makes you proud?
- What is one thing that you have learned in the past few weeks?
- What brings you joy and satisfaction in your work?
- What was a highpoint experience since we last met?
- Do you feel that you are using your greatest gifts/talents/strengths wisely?
- What are your most cherished values, and how are they reflected in your work?
- What were your earliest hopes and intentions as a nurse, and how have those changed over time?

Key #4: Embolden With Opportunity and Autonomy

"When I think about generativity," noted Todd G., "I think of letting go, letting others do it their way, and not trying to control everything." This aspect of generativity involves both the satisfaction and the struggle of loosening the reins of control and encouraging the next generation to exercise their own power and choices.

In granting autonomy, you may find yourself in a tug of war between your desire to invest in the next generation and your need to be needed (or to believe that "this place would fall apart without me"). Sandra J. confirms this problem and its resolution; she admits that letting go takes practice. "I remember when I first I went away and I was hysterical the whole week I was gone. Now, I turn the phone off when I go, and they are here, and I know it's all going to be here when I come back. Yes, because they need [to know how to survive]. What happens if I'm in a car accident tomorrow?"

And then, too, you may experience inner warfare about sustaining your stellar standards versus letting the team call the shots. This battle evokes the much-repeated rationale for micromanagement. ("I had to do it myself—because they won't do it as well as I would.")

Still, many leaders sidestep perfection and speak of the long-term dividends of training their staff to be independent of them. Marla B. spells out the benefits of giving the kids the keys to the car. "I don't feel like everything just goes to heck when I'm not there. I don't think twice if I'm not going to be there that they are going to be overstaffed or slacking off. But that comes from not pushing down their throats. It's really from giving them the autonomy and giving them respect and letting them be professional. [That] makes them want to do a professional job."

REFLECTION

Explore your resistance. What is holding you back from empowering your staff? Huber has described a leader's crucial pivot from delegation reluctance (driven by micromanagement, risk aversion, care taking, and the need to feel indispensable) to a practice of deliberate delegation grounded in trust and collaboration.[18]

....

....

....

....

....

Memo to lean-over-their-shoulder leaders: This shift is crucial. Because autonomy and generativity require that you delegate and share some of your authority and share power, accountability, and control.

How itchy do you feel at the prospect that a team member may not do it the way you would? Or be less than perfect?

....

....

....

....

....

What are gains and losses for you in making the shift that Huber described—increasing their motivation while decreasing your control?

....

....

....

....

....

Describe an experience when you emboldened your team to generate ideas or choose a means to complete a project or improve a quality metric.

....

....

....

....

....

Next, describe an experience where you were a leader with the plan—and the team's choices were not part of the conversation.

....

....

....

....

....

What would you want to teach other leaders about the difference in the outcomes?

....

....

....

....

....

EXPERIMENT

Nurse leader Ti King describes the process of giving staff responsibility and visibility as "provoking leadership."[19] Do a mental roll call of your team. Who might you ask to take your place or join you at a professional meeting? Become a champion or a first adapter of a quality or safety improvement? Craft a new policy? Continue their education? Conduct research or create a poster presentation? Take them out on a limb, but continue to check in with a light hand.

EXPERIMENT

Encourage the yet. Psychologist Carol Dweck suggests one word that defines a growth mindset and emboldens opportunity and autonomy: yet. As in, "I haven't learned how to do that, yet." "I haven't mastered that, yet." "I don't understand that, yet."[20] Convey the conviction that success is the child of consistent effort.

The generativity you have been exploring is a fruitful investment in the future of nursing—one that demands you remain alert and connected to your current team and to the generations to come.

Imagine a future where every conversation about succession planning or building leadership bench strength begins with stories of generativity in action. This storytelling would have the power to link past, present, and future and kindle creativity between the generations. It would affirm the agreement that there can be no succession planning without emotional investment.

Listen to how Mika S. addresses both her emotional and strategic intentions. "It is believing in the new generation's ability to care for me and my children as we age; to have the knowledge that my time in nursing was worth it. That I do leave, not only from this job, but from so many patients, that I can still remember back to by name, by sight, to know truly in my heart that I have made a positive difference. I am at the crux now of getting ready in succession planning to leave management and prepare others to want to step into this job."

Todd G. describes the circular dynamics of creative and linked generations at work. As he explains, "We are handing off responsibility. [At the same time] we are also taking from the generation in front of us throughout our entire career. I feel a sense of extreme obligation to carry on the legacy of the nurse leaders who are in front of me and not mess up what they accomplished, and also to create a more fertile ground for those nurses to come. It is a two-way street. We are simultaneously preparing ourselves and others for the future."

Todd's ideas about connecting the dots between generations reminded me of the wisdom of my father, Sam, who introduced me to generativity when I was a prickly teenager by explaining, "When you are growing up, you inherit the world from us. When you are older, we inherit the world from you."

Ask a Nurse Leader: Peer Wise Ideas About Generativity

Pick one or more of these examples of peer wisdom to explore.
What lessons from your own experience come to mind as you read these stories?

◇◇◇◇◇◇◇◇◇◇◇◇

"I find that the most rewarding time is when you see someone whom you have been mentoring into a lead position suddenly not need to ask any questions regarding their role as a leader. When they come to my office, it's not to ask how to do anything, but just to visit and let me know how things are going. They manage the department as if it is second nature. They have earned the respect from not only the staff and peers, but the surgeons, who can be very difficult to please."

Joan D.

Service Line Manager, OR/Anesthesia

◇◇◇◇◇◇◇◇◇◇◇◇

"The first couple of months into my new nurse manager role, I was approached by the chair of our unit-based council (UBC). The UBC is for staff members only; leadership was to take a step back and allow the group to create a vision for the unit and make positive changes. She asked if I could help her increase attendance to the UBC. In the past, only three of the same staff members would attend. She was grateful to these three, but knew if others were to attend that new ideas would be plentiful. But she didn't want the meeting to be one full of complaints; she wanted staff to use the time wisely and be productive. We sat together to brainstorm. I asked questions like, why do you think they do not attend? What changes have been made that others valued through this UBC? How do you see this working?

"We worked through an agenda together and discussed topics to be covered, but I also told her, if great ideas are generated and everyone is feeding off one another in a positive manner, you don't have to stick to the agenda; see where it takes you. She asked me to attend the next meeting to coach her through it. Ten staff members showed, so we already doubled the attendance. What came next is when I realized she was ready to take this on her own and I knew she would succeed.

"Before the next meeting, she came to me with the agenda. I asked if she wanted me there, but she said, 'I'm OK, I think I've got this.' The next day I saw her: She had a giant smile on her face. She was full of excitement and said 30 staff members attended the meeting. She started telling me of these team-based ideas, how staff were going to improve communication. She wanted an area of her own in the break room so that others could put topics to be discussed on the white board. She did her own minutes, created a communication tree, and notebook for the group.

"The UBC continues to be a success. This RN had it in her all along to lead her peers—that I knew. And she was thankful [to me] for helping find her inner leader, by not giving her my solutions, but allowing her to find them on her own—with some guidance, encouragement, and just a little nudge."

Kelle M.
Manager, Orthopedics

◇◇◇◇◇◇◇◇◇◇

"As far as my practice in generativity, I really rely on my past experiences with nurturing our next leaders. I have had plenty of unsuccessful attempts at promoting young leaders into roles that they were either not suited for or didn't have what it takes to make the cut. Most of the time, my thoughts were they had what it took for success, but it was a wild guess on my part. Over the past 2 years, my practice has changed to utilizing tools to assess personalities and strengths. I evaluate the person's contributions to committee work or volunteer events. And additionally, I strongly evaluate the person's passion for leadership. These few components of evaluations have allowed for more success stories with the growth of future leaders.

"In addition, I really like the color-coded personality test. I specifically look for employees I'm considering for promotion who test out Red or Blue. Red being a leader and blue being compassionate. We have had some recent turnover with a couple of nurse administrators, and I utilized this tool with a few of my internal candidates and it really seems to work. Unfortunately, human resources will not allow me to test any external candidates. In addition, last summer I cultured my annual employee evaluations around their personality trait. I found this to be a much more efficient way to connect to the employee, rather than taking the same approach to every employee. I was able to create action plans that would produce a more obtainable outcome for the employees, which saved me a lot of headaches! I plan on doing the same again this summer as well!"

Morgan T.
Manager, PICC Team Clinical Transition Unit

◇◇◇◇◇◇◇◇◇◇

"One of my happiest moments was when I returned to work yesterday after being away for a week at the AONE Nurse Manager Fellowship in New Orleans, Louisiana. My core group of charge nurses in the emergency department led with confidence and purpose, reinforcing the fact that they can do it without me! In addition to Ebola preparedness drills and preparation for transition to a new online documentation system, they faced a significant increase in patient volume, callouts due to illness, and an unexpected leave of absence. Each decision they made was carefully thought out and had our patients' best interest in mind. It brings me great joy to witness bedside nurses grow professionally!"

Lisa V.
Manager, Emergency Department

◇◇◇◇◇◇◇◇◇◇

"We utilize a shared governance concept in our busy MICU, where each staff member contributes in some way to our success through committee work or other unit/hospital involvement.

This helps prepare the next set of leaders in many ways, as they become increasingly involved in projects and take accountability for our success. In October our hospital was designated to be the only adult hospital in the state to handle in-patient Ebola patients. I was abruptly pulled out of my usual role as nurse manager and went full-time into planning the new unit. My assistant nurse manager and I discussed an action plan.

"We have always looked for ways to help emerging leaders take on new responsibilities, and we were able to tap into that resource to help with her increased workload. I had already begun teaching her how to do the monthly variance report and we always discuss disciplinary action and develop action plans together, so she was well-equipped to have crucial conversations on her own. She had developed good interview skills over time and was confident in taking the lead with this as well. She has always been deeply involved in collaborative relationships with our unit medical leaders, and easily took the lead in decision making in my absence.

"We talked several times each week about her challenges so I could coach and give advice. She grew immensely as a result of my lengthy absence and really found her own way of leading. Now that I'm back part time, it has been interesting negotiating our new roles. I feel like more of a visitor! I have tried to avoid reversing any decisions she has made and continue with the coaching role, asking her what help she needs. Watching her successfully take on some significant challenges with staffing, patient and family situations, and moving the unit forward from a leadership standpoint has been very gratifying.

"One of the most tangible pieces of evidence that our succession plan works is that our nosocomial complication rate stayed at extremely low levels—a function left completely to our nursing staff leaders to continually monitor. About 6 months prior to my absence, we had implemented a program where one of the staff evaluates all patients designated as high risk (three or more devices in place, such as central line, ventilator, feeding tube …) every shift. They review a checklist of nursing standards of care and ensure all standards are met in each room. This takes the load off of busy staff members, who may just not have time to change that central dressing or turn their patient again. Our data has been very compelling and we did not lose one bit of momentum in my absence! I am very proud of everyone on our team! They do amazing work."

Cheryl M.
Manager, ICU

◇◇◇◇◇◇◇◇◇◇◇

"I have a relatively new charge nurse who has only been a nurse for about 3 years. She has expressed some uneasiness or anxiousness with performing the charge role as she doesn't always seem prepared for every situation. I have been coaching her and providing feedback as events come up. Today, she had a couple issues present themselves. While not clinical in nature, she handled them exactly as she should and was on top of everything. The first issue was a toilet back-up in a semi-private room. Both patients needed to be out of the room while the toilet was removed. Without prompting, she called the house supervisor, alerted her of the situation and that both patients were to be discharged today. When the rooms came empty she called plant ops, the house sup, and housekeeping to arrange the repair and post-cleaning. A simple task, but she was very confident as she told, already did that. It is great to see nurses grow clinically but also take ownership of the unit and their role."

Beth T.
Manager, Comprehensive and Medical Progressive Care Unit

◇◇◇◇◇◇◇◇◇◇

"When I think about generativity, I think of letting go, letting others do it their way, and not trying to control everything. The other aspect is that as we are handing off we are also taking on from the generation in front of us throughout our entire career.

"I feel a sense of extreme obligation to carry on the legacy of the nurse leaders who are in front of me and not mess up what they accomplished, and only create a more fertile ground for nursing in the future … for those to come. It is a two-way street. We are simultaneously preparing others and ourselves for the future.

"A key component of generativity is not waiting for the next generation to be the drivers of evolution. We must be reborn continuously as we reinvent ourselves internally, creating new generations of ourselves."

Todd G.
Director, Critical Care Services

◇◇◇◇◇◇◇◇◇◇

"There is no denying that our roles have increased in scope. In the operating room, we have adapted efficiency initiatives directed toward meeting metrics such as first case starts and turnover times. This is a part of an OR optimization project that revised our policies on surgery scheduling, block management, preference card management, and surgical case preparation. The roles of the staff were modified and parallel processing between staff and physicians was established.

"A major component in ensuring the success of the optimization project is transparency. I prepare a daily report on delays in turnover time based on an established surgical service specific goal. This report is sent to all surgical service chairpersons, surgeons, anesthesia providers, and nursing staff involved in cases that had a delay. I used to be the only person responsible for preparing and sending this daily turnover delay report, as well as investigating clarifications from physicians regarding the delay reasons indicated by the circulator. During the last few months, our assistant nurse manager has assumed this extensive and sometimes difficult role. I say extensive because the task summarized the person's understanding of the entire optimization process. The assistant charge nurse and I engage the physicians, staff, and support services daily to discuss the delay reasons associated with their case(s). This requires in-depth knowledge of the processes to remain consistent and objective in addressing the questions raised by staff and physicians.

"I also started taking one of our assistant nurse managers and service coordinators to our health system leadership monthly meeting. During this meeting, ongoing projects, financial status (monthly and YTD), reimbursements, payer mix, readmission rates, labor cost, patient satisfaction scores, and our reported HACs, to mention a few, are presented to all the managers, directors, and assistant vice presidents of both the health system and enterprise. I believe that attending these meetings helps improve their understanding of the current health care environment and our institution's actions to adapt to the new reality. Their understanding in turn will affect their management skills and serve as a resource when they share this information and understanding of the institution's goals with the staff and physicians. The information they will share and decisions that they make will have more far-reaching influence than I can present in a weekly staff meeting."

Ri D.
Manager, OR

◇◇◇◇◇◇◇◇◇◇

"A time when I gave an emerging leader the keys to lead was: Having a new clinical nurse leader on unit, new role to the organization and her new to the organization. It was difficult to find a project that I felt she could succeed with, alone, in a relatively short of amount of time. I reflected back on the qualities that led us, myself and the staff, to hire her on, and let that be the guide and trust. Our CNL took over restructuring our 40-bed med surg multidisciplinary care rounds from tabletop discussion with one RN at a time coming in to present her patients, which was lengthy, to driving those care rounds to be at the bedside! She presented the idea to me with pros/cons and asked for support. I fully supported and RNs and the multidisciplinary bought in.

"Now the staff could not imagine care rounds any other way. The RN stays in close proximity to patient, diagnostics, and the team can engage in rapid bedside assessment and dialogue with patient, family, and RN while still cutting rounds to less than an hour."

Anabel B.
Patient Care Manager, Surgical Service Line

◇◇◇◇◇◇◇◇◇◇

"I manage a 42-bed general surgery, urology, plastics, bariatric with 16-bed telemetry in a large teaching institution. My unit is part of a surgical cluster including an 18-bed neuro trauma unit, which recently lost the nurse manager, 12-bed surgical trauma, 24-bed vascular unit, and 26-bed transplant unit. In the past, I managed the surgical trauma unit while they searched for a new manager. One day last December, my director approached me and asked if I would consider taking on the interim nurse manager [role] for the 18-bed neuro trauma unit, along with my 42-bed unit. The effective date being after the holidays. I had about two weeks to plan. I always look at a challenge as an opportunity but knew little about the staff or unit, and there would be no handoff from the previous nurse manager! I truly believe that the success of a team is its ability to function well in the absence of their leader. Now was the time to put that belief into action.

"So I looked to four of my potential leaders among my nursing staff and asked for their input. I discussed my additional role in managing the ICU and that I needed to be more visible on that unit but still maintain the daily operations for my current surgical unit. We had just completed the roll out of patient progression rounds in the hospital led by the nurse manager and case coordinator. The staff (who I believe always have the answers) developed the following plan:

1. The four nurses would adjust their schedules so they would consistently be resource for the unit.
2. They would start the shift with one less patient in their assignment so they could lead the patient progression rounds.
3. After 11 a.m., they would add one more patient to their assignment.
4. They would run morning huddle and ensure consistent communication to the next shift.
5. They would manage daily operations of staffing and patient throughput.

"Of note, our unit at any given time could discharge 10 to 16 patients and then turn around and get the same amount of postoperative patients in a 12-hour day.

"Well, my interim position lasted for 9 months, and during that time, I was never so proud of my team on my surgical team. Not only did they maintain stability on the unit, but I noticed that in the event they were out, another nurse (not part of the original four) took on the resource role and led progression rounds in the same way as their peers. As I reflect upon those 9 months, I was successful in my interim role because of those four nurses on my surgical unit.

"The best advice I could give a new nurse leader using this example is to always look for the potential leaders on your staff, making sure you mentor and educate them. You need to be prepared for unexpected opportunities in the constantly changing environment of health care."

Susanne Y.
Manager, ICU and surgery units

Your Thoughts?

Pick one or more of these examples of peer wisdom about generativity to explore.
What lessons from your own experiences come to mind as you read these stories?

....

....

....

....

....

Q & Q: Quote and Question

Consider each quote about *generativity* and answer the follow-up question from your own experience.

> Q: "The delicate balance of mentoring someone is not creating them in your own image but giving them the opportunity to create themselves."
>
> **Steven Spielberg**

Q: How do you balance passing on what you have learned and created with encouraging a new generation to discover and create?

....

....

....

....

> Q: "Spoon feeding in the long run teaches us nothing but the shape of the spoon."
>
> **E. M. Forster**

Q: How does this observation relate to your practice of generativity?

....

....

....

....

> Q: "Your most important task as a leader is to teach people how to think and ask the right questions so that the world doesn't go to hell if you take a day off."
>
> **Jeffrey Pfeffer**

Q: What are you doing to teach your team to lead so that the unit doesn't descend into chaos on your days off?

....

....

....

....

> Q: "If there is any responsibility in the cycle of life it must be that one generation owes to the next that strength by which it can come to face ultimate concerns in its own way."
>
> **Erik Erickson**

Q: What are the strengths you are developing in your team members—so that they can meet their concerns in their own way?

....

....

....

....

> Q: "If you light the path for someone it will also brighten your own path."
>
> **Buddhist proverb**

Q: Can you describe a time when your acts of generativity—growing new leaders—brightened your own path as a leader?

....

....

....

....

> Q: "A mentor is someone who sees more talent and ability within you, than you see in yourself, and helps bring it out of you."
>
> **Bob Proctor**

Q: **Can you recall someone whose acts of generativity brought out more talent and ability in you than you saw in yourself? Have you applied these actions in your own practice?**

....

....

....

....

Deep Dive Resources: Generativity

Books

de St. Aubin, E., & McAdams, D. P. (Eds.). (2004). *The generative society: Caring for future generations.* American Psychological Association.

Grossman, S. (2013). *Mentoring in nursing.* Springer.

Killhallon, K., & Thomson, J. (2012). *Mentoring in nursing and healthcare.* Wiley.

Kotre, J. (1996). *Outliving the self. Generativity and the interpretation of lives.* Norton. (Free download available at http://books.google.com/books?id=hUQ0ZgWfiIMC&printsec=frontcover&dq=out-living+the+self#v=onepage&q&f=false)

Kotre, J. (1999). *Make it count: How to generate a legacy that gives meaning to your life.* Free Press.

McAdams, D. P., & de St. Aubin, E. (Eds.). (1998). *Generativity and adult development; how and why we care for the next generation.* American Psychological Association.

Porter O'Grady, T., & Malloch, K. (2015). *The career handoff: A health care leader's guide to knowledge as wisdom transfer across the generations.* Sigma Tau International.

Vance, C. (2005). Leader as mentor. In H. R. Feldman & M. J. Greenberg (Eds.), *Educating nurses for leadership* (pp. 80–97). Springer Publishing Company.

Zachary, L. (2005). *Creating a mentoring culture.* Jossey Bass.

Professional Journals

Anderson, C. (2000). Our obligation to the next generation. *Nursing Outlook, 48*(4), 149–150.

Bally, J. (2007). The role of nursing leadership in creating a mentoring culture in acute care environments. *Nursing Economics, 25*(3), 143.

Beckmann Murray, R. (2002). Mentoring. Perceptions of the process and its significance. *Journal of Psychosocial Nursing, 40*(4), 44–51.

Block, L. M., Claffey, C., Korow, M. K., & McCaffrey, C. (2005). The value of mentorship within nursing organizations. *Nursing Forum, 40*(4), 134–140.

Doerwald, F., Zacher, H., Van Yperen, N. W., & Scheibe, S. (2021). Generativity at work: A meta-analysis. *Journal of Vocational Behavior, 125.*

Ghislieri, C., & Gatti, P. (2012). Generativity and balance in leadership. *Leadership, 8*(3), 257–275.

Jackson, D. (2008). Random acts of guidance: Personal reflections on professional generosity. *Journal of Clinical Nursing, 17*(20), 269–270.

Linderman, A., Pesut, D., & Disch, J. (2015). Sense making and knowledge transfer: Capturing the knowledge and wisdom of nursing leaders. *Journal of Professional Nursing, 31*(4), 290–297.

McAdams, D. (2001). Generativity: The new definition of success. *Spirituality and Health,* 26–33.

Parse, R. R. (2002). Mentoring moments. *Nursing Science Quarterly, 15*(2), 97.

Video

TEDx. (2016, April). *Bogdan Gogu: Why curiosity and mentorship will change your life* [Video]. YouTube. https://youtu.be/ibyvpjukl38

Figure Credit

Change Agility

Address the Challenge of the New

"Change is frightening. Change is stressful. Change is difficult. Change will never happen. Change happens too often. Change is too expensive.

"As nurse managers we hear these statements from our staff, our peers, our patients, and sometimes from the little voice inside ourselves. This year I stopped listening to these statements, took a chance on change, and it paid off!"

◇◇◇◇◇◇◇◇◇◇◇◇◇◇◇◇◇◇

Nurse leaders are expected to be the change whisperers in their organizations. You are the ones who talk and walk your team through change and inspire their innovations. As your colleague explains, this role demands that you understand that change is an emotional as well as procedural issue.

The plot thickens with a supervisor who peppers you with questions of how and when you can deliver the change—and who may be exasperated by the emotional messiness of change—asking you, "Why can't they just get on with it?"

In this laboratory, we will explore how to address both feelings and strategy to energize and mobilize both you and your team to "take a chance on change that pays off." Our working definition of change leadership defines you as a coach who nurtures your team's capacity to address changes and integrate new learning or practices.[1] We explore this idea knowing that you will also need to develop an inner coach. Because change also whispers to you.

Social scientists and songwriters of every stripe have described these emotional and procedural aspects of change. As noted earlier, psychologist Daniel Goleman explains the difference by describing the brain's response to change as an epic battle between your amygdala and your cerebral cortex.[2] When you are stressed by feelings about change, your amygdala, the brain's stress detector, takes over. Your body is flooded with stress hormones to prepare for emergency. As a result, your cerebral cortex, the problem-solving part of the brain, shuts down.

A brilliant lesson in this brainy battle comes from leadership sages Andrew Grashow, Ronald Heifetz and Marty Linsky, who explore the difference between technical changes—say, reorganizing a work area—and adaptive changes, like switching to bedside reporting.[3] A technical change can be accomplished with a quick and easy solution. Adaptive change can require new learning, asks us to unpack our habits and to experience uncertainty and perhaps a time of self-doubt and loss.

The biggest failure of leadership, they warn, is treating all changes as technical ones. Because adaptive change can demand that people question and perhaps adapt aspects of their identity, it also challenges their sure-footed sense of competence.[4]

Tom R., who designed an innovative time-saving technology for his team, discovered the difference. "I put all my energy and planning into classes and tutorials to prepare my team for the change. When they resisted, I realized I also needed to talk about their feelings—their concerns and insecurities—about using the new system."

Adaptive change is the subject of musicians, from Bob Dylan to Beyoncé, who chronicle change in their lives. Just listen to iconic rocker David Bowie's anthem to change, whose stuttering chorus of "ch- ch- ch- changes" urges us "to turn and face the strange."[5] The practice of change leadership involves toggling between facing the emotions of the unfamiliar and managing the procedural issues that drive change agility and innovation.

REFLECTION

Describe three recent changes in your organization. Are they technical changes (quick and easy solutions) or adaptive changes (may require new learning or changes in values, roles, relationships, accountability, and approaches to work)?

1. ....

....

....

....

2. ....

....

....

....

3. ....
....
....
....
....

As you coach your team, your past experiences will influence your approach to change.
Write a brief bulleted change autobiography. List childhood and young adult changes (a new school, home, or job). Note emotional aspects of these changes.

....
....
....
....
....

Consider and describe your parents, teachers, preceptors, and supervisors as change leaders. What strategies and emotions did they model in guiding your family or team through change?

....
....
....
....
....

Four Key Ideas for Change Leadership

Keep these past and current change challenges in mind as your consider four key ideas of change leadership. Continue to reflect on your experiences; compare your theories of change with the ones that follow. Identify your best practices and plan to experiment with some new actionable strategies.

Key	Strategies	Your best practices
Key #1 Acknowledge and legitimize feelings.	~Explore resistance. ~Appraise level of trust. ~Nurture psychological safety. ~Recognize endings.	
Key #2 Align change with purpose.	~Underline the why. ~Strike up the brand. ~Highlight shared values. ~Discover competing commitments.	
Key #3 Encourage agency by offering genuine choices.	~Offer genuine choices. ~Get an early start. ~Try small tests of change. ~Describe change style. ~Suggest question storming.	
Key #4 Craft a solution-focused approach.	~Turn complaints into commitments. ~Pose affirmative rather than deficit questions. ~Use positive expectancy.	

EXPERIMENT

Feel the change. Pick up a pen and write for 1 minute in this space about your response to a recent change at work.

....

....

....

....

....

Now, change your pen to your other hand and continue writing for another minute.

....

....

....

....

....

Observe your responses: Smart but feeling dumb? Wanting to hide your work? Frustrated about not meeting your standards?

....

....

....

....

....

How can this exercise inform your response when your team pushes back about change?

....

....

....

....

....

Let's start by kicking three change clichés to the curb. "It is what it is" (the perfect discussion/motivation shut-up ploy). "The only constant is change" (a platitude that offers neither comfort nor courage). "Someday you will laugh at this." (The only response to this nonstarter is, Can you give me an exact date?) These clichés are empty because they fail to distinguish between technical and adaptive change. They ignore four key leadership practices of change leadership: acknowledgement of feelings, alignment with purpose, encouragement of agency, and framing a problem-solving outlook.

Compare these clichés with the modus operandi of Cheryl M., who manages a rapidly changing MICU using these practices: "We begin prepping staff for the change as soon as we know it will occur. We are transparent about the changes and challenges facing us and adjusting to those changes. We discuss their fears and potential barriers openly."

She explains, "When we changed to bar-coded medication administration, we related it to general safety practices and how bar coding could have caught some of our past medication errors. All changes are brought to the staff through shared governance and staff meetings to discuss the change, assess the barriers, and get the staff engaged in creating the change their way."

Key #1: Acknowledge and Legitimize Feelings
Like Cheryl M., a change leader's agenda puts acknowledgment and management of feelings ahead of flow charts and benchmarks. This priority is highlighted in research conducted by Mel Fugate and Angelo Kinicki, who detail the dangers of "escape coping," where an

overload of thoughts and emotions drive actions to avoid the difficulties of change.[6] For instance, a member of your team announces he is "too busy" to attend training classes for a new medical records system.

Creating an atmosphere of trust—one where feelings can be openly expressed—is a crucible in leading your team through challenging changes. Find guidance in teamwork expert Nick Lencioni's definition of trust: the confidence among team members that their peer's intentions are good and members can be *vulnerable* around each other.[7]

Psychological safety is the phrase leadership scholar Amy Edmondson uses to describe this kind of vulnerability.[8] With a sense of safety, your team members are more willing to admit weaknesses, skill deficiencies, and interpersonal shortcomings. They are able to ask for help and to be confident that this will not be used against them.

REFLECTION

Describe a work setting where you experienced a sense of psychological safety. What were the actions and attitudes of team members and leadership that contributed to this feeling?

....

....

....

....

....

REFLECTION

Assess the level of psychological safety your team experiences. Are they able to ask each other for help or express their worries and be confident that their vulnerabilities will not be held against them?

....

....

....

....

....

Take the time to name and recognize the thoughts and feelings of your team, whose attitudes may range from complacency ("We have always done it this way") to unspoken concerns ("What if I can't do this?"), and from grief ("I miss the way we used to …") to anger ("Why didn't you ask *us*?").

You can begin by acknowledging the feelings that resist procedure: a learning curve that causes nosebleeds, more accountability and complexity, a longer to-do list, confusion or lack of confidence about benefits. Next, give them a wide berth to express the reluctance that reveals why change is unwelcome: Familiarity creates comfort and a sure-footed confidence.

Tanya S. expressed frustration about a group of ED nurses who, despite extensive training, are resisting an IV conversion. "They have gone so far as to hoard old supplies, to struggle and be dissatisfied."

Tanya's situation is reminder of the need to provide your team with emotional support when a change undermines their confidence or sense of purpose.[9] Nurse leaders Mags Balfour and Charlotte Clarke have highlighted how tempting it is to revert back to familiar ways of working once the team leader driving the change moves on.[10] They suggest that change engagement and sustainment requires nurses to find value in the new ways of working. If Tanya looks behind the hide and seek, she will understand that it may be difficult for her team to value a new way of working with this new equipment if they lack confidence, or feel concerned about putting patients at risk.

REFLECTION

Consider these three statements of resistance to change. What are the emotions behind each one?

"This is too complicated."

....

....

....

....

....

"We don't have the staff."

....

....

....

....

....

"What was wrong with the way we/I have been doing this?"

....

....

....

....

....

EXPERIMENT

Ask for an analogy. Take a fast track to discover your own feelings or those of your team by asking, "What does this change remind me of?" This lighter approach allows you to explore the emotional content of each comparison. Review your/their choices. What are the emotions they evoke?

Acknowledgment by Analogy

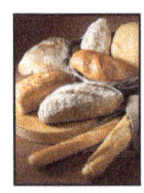

This change reminds me of _____ (animal)

This change reminds me of _____ (bread)

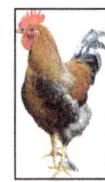

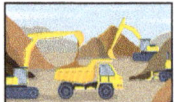

This change reminds me of _____ (movie)

This change reminds me _____ (vehicle)

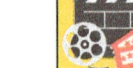

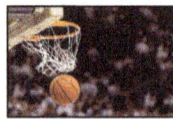

This change reminds me of _____ (song)

This change reminds me of _____ (sport)

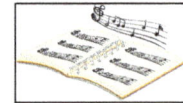

FIGURE 6.1

EXPERIMENT

Recognize endings. Poet T. S. Eliot offered advice about the acknowledgment of loss when he observed, "What we call the beginning is often the end. And to make an end is to make a beginning. The end is where we start from."[11]

You can enhance the meaning of endings with what sociologist Sarah Lawrence-Lightfoot calls "rituals of good-bye."[12] This can be simple statements of what you and team will miss or a cake and cookies ceremony when closing one unit and moving to a new one.

Key #2: Align Change With Purpose

Underline the why.[13] Focus your team on the line of sight between a specific change and their bigger-picture purpose as health care providers. Dorothy H. describes this alignment: "We give lots of information, but we connect the dots and align the compelling reasons and values that are underlined in the change."

Moving from the details to the bigger picture of purpose is key to engagement in change. Margaret L., who led her staff through several much-lamented office moves, observes, "What seems to help us make these changes more readily is to keep the patient in mind with the common goal for what will support the patient best. This focus helps us to make better decisions and to forge through difficulties."

REFLECTION

Describe a projected change in your organization. Imagine describing this change to your team. Create a juicy statement that highlights purpose and shared values—one that underlines the why along with the what.

Use action verbs: enhance, manage, elevate, improve, reduce, increase.

REFLECTION

Change leaders John Kotter and Dan Cohen suggest that the key to aligning change with purpose is drilling down to the details and the destination.[14] Build on conveying the purpose of the change you just described to your team by answering a trio of questions:

What are the plans and strategies?

....

....

....

....

Where will they take us?

....

....

....

....

Why do we want to be there?

....

....

....

....

....

 EXPERIMENT

Strike up the brand. Engage the we-never-did-it-this-way-before bunch with an appeal to brand identity. Link the change to a core value of your team or organization. You might say, "No, we have not used bar coding for medication in the past. But we have always set the gold standard for patient safety. Bar coding can help us catch errors earlier."

In their essential book, *Immunity to Change*, psychologists Robert Kegan and Lisa Laskow-Lahey urge us to examine our ambivalence about change—our "competing commitments."[15] They invite us to name the hidden fears and assumptions that cause us to drive change with one foot on the gas and the other on the brakes.

For example, you may be committed to establishing leadership rounds as a way of enhancing patient care. At the same time, you also are committed to having your director or CNO review your units with stars in her eyes. Your fear is that the feedback from patients and families will detract from your unit's stellar image.

REFLECTION

Kegan and Laskow-Lahey suggest that when you argue with your ambivalence, you can refocus your line of sight to the purpose and the execution of the change. Think of a situation where you are ambivalent about change. Map out your competing commitments and the fear that drives them. What did you discover? How might this idea assist you when dealing with resistance on your team?

I am committed to the purpose or value of …	What am I doing that prevents my commitment from being realized?	I might also be committed to …	My fear is that …

Key #3: Encourage Agency by Offering Genuine Choices

Beware of commands disguised as choices. Imagine that you receive an email asking for feedback about moving decentralized telemetry to a centralized location. Then, before you can respond, you find out that this change has already been approved. To avoid this bait-and-switch approach with your team, you must be transparent in naming changes and innovations that are non-negotiable.

Motivational psychologists Edward Deci and Richard Ryan anchor their work in the power of self-determination and urge leaders to offer "autonomy support."[16] The role of choice in change lies in discovering and introducing aspects of the change that you and your team can control. As one manager explained, "We may have to change, but how we do it is up to the staff."

Denise W., who led her staff in a quality improvement and efficiency process in their working space, explains how her offer of agency was linked to positive outcomes: "I think what helped is that we empowered the staff who worked in the area to make the decisions of how the unit looked and where equipment, supplies, etc., should be placed."

REFLECTION

Describe a projected innovation or change in your organization. Consider which aspects are set in concrete and which might be open to choice. Can you offer your team choices about who? How? When?

....

....

....

....

....

EXPERIMENT

Unwrap small packages. Early wins and small tests of change are the currency of agency. Quality improvement innovators like Edward Deming have crafted the widely used PDSA (plan-do-study-act) model.[17] The completion of each cycle leads directly into the start of the next cycle.

In this model, a team learns from each small test. What worked and what didn't work? What should be kept, changed, or filed in the circular file? How can we use the new knowledge to plan the next test? The team continues to refine the change as needed. Linking small tests of change helps overcome a group or individual's initial resistance to change. Staff and colleagues will be more willing to road-test a small change if they know the direction can be modified.

EXPERIMENT

Trial the change. Erik M. wanted to increase the number of visitors allowed in the room in an ICU. His approach: "I shared our logic behind expanding visitation and told staff we would 'trial' the change. I let them know that we would be tracking issues that arose, and if the cons began to outweigh the pros that we would change back. I think knowing that we would track issues and that the change wasn't set in stone helped ease some of the angst."

EXPERIMENT

Start question storming. Turn brainstorming upside down and ask your team for questions instead of suggestions. This tool, described in *The Innovator's DNA* by thought leaders Jeff Dyer, Hal Gregerson, and Clayton Christensen, maps a low-risk way for them to interact with—and experience a sense of agency about—projected changes.[18]

Here is the drill: Describe a projected change or innovation. Make sure it is a pending change and not a fait acompli. Divide into groups of four to six. Start by posing every possible question about adapting to this change. Write every question down. Encourage silly and off-the-wall and wild questions. Do not judge, censor, or discuss any of the questions (volume is the goal). Stop after 10 to 25 questions. Pick five top-priority questions to explore.

EXPERIMENT

Consider each team member's change style. Change researchers Chris Musselwhite and Randell Jones describe a continuum of three preferences in working with change, and underlines the contribution of each preference.[19] Consider what each member brings and how to approach them and leverage their preference. Increase their sense of agency and self-awareness by asking them to describe themselves in terms of these preferences. Note that each style brings something to the table of change.

Conservers prefer to stay the course and would wait till it breaks to fix it. They can cope with change step by step, and contribute by asking the hard questions. *Pragmatists* will do what is necessary and prefer change that is linked to common goals; they help the team see both sides of an argument. *Originators* get squirmy with the status quo and enjoy expansive change, risk, and uncertainty; they urge the team to challenge assumptions.

Key #4: Craft a Solution-Focused Approach

Emma T. has been very successful in creating a climate of psychological safety with her team. Yet she wonders, Can there be too much of a good thing? As she explained, "My team are very safe in expressing their feelings, but how do I keep my huddles from turning into a complaining session?"

If Emma sent you an email or met you for coffee to ask about her team, what advice would you give?

....

....

....

....

....

Consider your suggestions alongside two related methodologies that also offer answers to Emma's question. The solution-focused approach[20] and appreciative inquiry[21] emphasize desired outcomes rather than deficits or problem descriptions; they appreciate successes rather than stumbles.

Solution-focused practice has its roots in a coaching and consulting model of the 1980s developed by therapist Steve de Shazer et al.,[22] and in the work of anthropologist Gregory Bateson.[23]

EXPERIMENT

Study the scale. Leadership consultant Madeline Duclos suggests that a solution-focused conversation might begin with a simple question of scaling: "On a scale from 0 to 10, how effective have you been in this project?" If your team member says "six," you then ask, "What are the main successes that have led you to climb to that number?"[24]

Solution-focused approaches have been translated into actionable strategies for leadership and organizational change[25] and discussed in the work of psychologists like Robert Kegan and Lisa Laskow-Lahey.[26]

Let's return to Emma's dilemma. Above all, she is asking for a way to avoid the coffee kvetch—to shift her team from describing problems to discussing solutions. Her challenge suggests that turning complaints into commitments is the most nuanced balancing act of being a change coach.

Kegan and Laskow-Lahey's cheeky and strategic descriptions of workplace communication have nicknamed on-the-job complaints as BMW (bitching, moaning, and whining). Still, they see complaints as camouflage; behind every complaint there is an idea or belief that a person cares about. Otherwise, why would they be upset?

For example, recall the ER nurses who complained and resisted using the new IV equipment. They were also expressing a commitment to doing the job well and a desire (and fear) about keeping patients from harm.

The key in understanding their hide and seek is to find the commitment or value disguised in the complaint. Because if team members can stop thinking of themselves as complainers, and begin to think of themselves as people who are committed to something, they are walking in the direction of solutions.

 REFLECTION

Invite yourself or your team to consider several leading questions, adapted from Kegan and Laskow-Lahey.

What kinds of support would help me in meeting the challenge of this change?

....

....

....

....

....

What is one thing I feel strongly about during this change process? Complete the following sentence: "I am committed to the value or the importance of ..."

....

....

....

....

....

Consider your participation. What am I doing (or not doing) that prevents my commitment/value from being fully realized? Do I have competing values commitments?

....

....

....

....

....

The widely applied practice of appreciative inquiry, introduced in the work of David Cooperrider and Suresh Srivastva, began with a study and appreciation of the strengths of the storied Cleveland Clinic.[27] This practice has been applied in a variety of health care settings.[28, 29] In their approach, words create worlds and the questions we ask determine the solutions we find.

They urge change coaches to begin by asking appreciative affirmative questions (What is working? What do we want more of?) rather than downer deficit queries (What is wrong? Why isn't this working?).

In this framework, the question, How can we stop all of the noise in the ER? becomes, How can we create a more restful healing environment for our patients? Instead of asking, Why does my team keep hoarding the old IV supplies? you would ask, How can we work together to help the team feel comfortable and competent with new process/product?

REFLECTION

Rewrite each of these deficit questions to craft an appreciative affirmative question—one that will guide the team to a solution.

Deficit question: How do we change our overwhelming and inconsistent discharge process?

Appreciative affirmative question:

....

....

....

....

....

Deficit question: Why is there a breakdown in communication during shift changes?

Appreciative affirmative question:

....

....

....

....

....

EXPERIMENT

Appreciative inquiry practice suggests that actions are partly based on what we imagine, expect, or anticipate. You can fast-forward by trying a thought experiment. Imagine that it is 2 months from now. The change you have struggled to adapt to has become "the way we do things around here." Then ask:

What positive outcomes will we be able to see?

....

....

....

....

....

What is one small change that might have made this possible?

....

....

....

....

....

How were we able to overcome the feeling of one change too many?

....

....

....

....

....

What other actions could have contributed to the success of creating this change?

....

....

....

....

....

Think of a current change or innovation in your organization. How might a solution-focused approach or an appreciative inquiry tool enable your team to adapt to change—integrate new conditions, practices, or processes?

....

....

....

....

....

With every step or strategy, change leaders can coach their teams with a spirit of openness, curiosity, and self-compassion. Two wise nurse leaders light the path. Tonya H. describes the graceful attitude. "It is important to remain curious, be open to change, be flexible and agile, and be willing to forgive self and others." And Cynthia J. sums up the mission: "We need to understand the importance of our role as innovators. Embrace risk taking and small tests of change that support safe, timely, efficient, effective, equitable, and patient-centered care. Find joy in small things."

Ask a Nurse Leader: Peer Wise Ideas About Change Agility

Pick one or more of these examples of peer wisdom to explore.
What lessons from your own experience come to mind as you read these stories?

◇◇◇◇◇◇◇◇◇◇

"Change is frightening. Change is stressful. Change is difficult. Change will never happen. Change happens too often. Change is too expensive. As nurse managers, we hear these statements from our staff, our peers, our patients, and sometimes from the little voice inside ourselves. This year I stopped listening to these statements, took a chance on change, and it paid off!

"Our hospital did not have a designated intermediate care unit, and there was a definite need as ICU beds became an increasingly scarce resource. There were patients being admitted to the ICU that could be cared for in an intermediate care unit, if one existed. My staff and I embarked on a plan to transition the CT/vascular unit to become the first intermediate care unit in the hospital. The staff already possessed advanced skills, so I knew they were the perfect group to take on this challenge.

"The patient care facilitator on the unit is an advanced practice nurse with many years of experience and who the staff, physicians, leadership, and I admire and respect. He became the champion for the project, and I was grateful for his ongoing support. I learned that frequent, thorough, and consistent communication was the key to keeping all participants engaged. Collecting data and sharing it with hospital leadership provided evidence that the changes we were making were positively impacting patient care.

"Perhaps the most important thing I learned this year is to believe in myself. I now have the confidence to cope with and successfully navigate change. I am happy and proud to report that we completed the 6-month pilot and officially opened on September 1!"

Dell R.
Manager, Cardiothoracic Surgery

◇◇◇◇◇◇◇◇◇◇

"I work for a dynamic MICU and health system where change is the norm. Over my 6 years as the nurse manager we have introduced new cardiac monitors, a new nurse call system, bar code medication administration, a new computer documentation system and upgrades, to name a few. For these types of changes, we arrange for training, we engage staff as champions—we provide them with extra training and make sure they are scheduled without patients during implementation to support the staff.

"Our leadership team also functions in this supportive role when we roll out new technology—we make sure we have time to be available to support the staff. We begin prepping staff for the change as soon as we know it will occur. We discuss their fears and potential barriers openly. All changes are brought to the staff through shared governance and staff meetings to discuss the change, assess the barriers, and get the staff engaged in creating the change their way. We may have to change, but how we do it is up to the staff.

"Recently we began inviting significant others to participate in our change of shift handoffs. This generated a lot of concern among the nurses, even though families routinely attended interdisciplinary rounds. We let them talk about their fears and worked through how we might handle those worst-case scenarios. We discussed the benefits of providing the family with the information they crave and the relationship building they need to feel comfortable with the care of their loved ones. We encouraged early adopters to discuss their experience and continue to role model this behavior.

"Perhaps the biggest change we've implemented in my unit is patient/family-centered care. We went from strict visiting hours and limits to open visitation. This culture change required a vision—a vision that we would treat all patients and families like we would want to be treated if we were the patient or family. A vision that we could individualize care and liberalize "rules" without inviting chaos. That we could empower our staff and charge nurses to decide what was reasonable behavior and to intervene where needed to control crowds, children, or inappropriate behavior. That one size did not fit all. Including families in inter-disciplinary rounds was part of this change. We spent a lot of time working with staff that were not used to having families at the bedside 24-7. This meant staff meetings to address concerns and assist with communication skills and individualizing limits. Assuring we would support them when needed. Being there to assist in the change 24-7. Working through what went wrong. Coaching individual staff who struggled with communication styles, at times assisting them in addressing the issue with families.

"We established regular leadership rounds where the nurse manager and/or assistant nurse manager meet all patients and/or families within the course of the week to determine if their expectations are met, communication is good between nurses and physicians, how we could better individualize their care or meet their needs. Ninety-nine percent of the feedback is excellent and this is shared with the staff weekly. In situations where there were communication gaps, staff are given the feedback and expectations are clear. Support is provided through coaching and/or other avenues as needed.

"We have also worked on teamwork on the unit. We have changed the culture from one of eating our young to one that is supportive and based on teamwork. Staff were once afraid to confront each other and routinely triangulated the leadership into their conflicts. Alter-natively, they would just live with an untenable situation until they burned out or broke down. We counseled staff on competent communication techniques, sent them to class, and mediated conflicts where they needed the assistance. We have gotten human resources and EPA involved as needed. We have made our expectations clear: bullying, gossiping, com-plaining are not acceptable. We address these problem behaviors with the parties, discuss expectations for appropriate communication, and investigate where the miscommunication and resentment are coming from. This has been successful over time. Negative staff have begun getting the message and are encouraged to seek more fulfilling positions (and many have done so).

"Staying transparent is important to keep in mind when guiding change!

"We are transparent about the changes and challenges facing us in health care today and how our health system is addressing or adjusting to those changes. For instance, we have talked about changes in reimbursement and how meaningful use affects us, and what technological changes are occurring to adjust for those requirements (bar coding). We also related bar coding to general safety practices and how bar coding could have caught some of our past medication errors. Our organization uses a 'blueprint for quality' that guides us as we implement changes. For instance, patient- and family-centered care is one imperative. We do relate changes, such as including the family in shift report, back to the blueprint initiative.

"I think part of culture change lies in who you hire as well. We have carefully recruited staff over the years. We spend quite a bit of time discussing teamwork, conflict resolution, and communication style with them during the interview. This also applies to patient- and family-centered care attitudes. We explore these attitudes and behaviors in depth as well. These are make or break responses for us. We have turned away outstanding nurses because we felt they lacked communication skills or ability to function well as a team."

Cheryl M.

Manager, Medical Intensive Care Unit

◇◇◇◇◇◇◇◇◇◇

"Professionally, I am in the midst of a change in the units I manage. I currently have two large general medicine units that are housed on the fourth floor and ninth floor. [This is a] very complex patient population, with the majority being drug and alcohol withdrawal. There was a small 14-bed medicine unit (4–6) that opened temporarily to accommodate the high census here at Yale. My director approached me and asked if I would give up my ninth-floor unit and take on the small 14-bed unit in addition to my fourth-floor unit (4–7). Geographically, this would put me on both units on the fourth floor, which was very appealing to me. However, it was a tough decision. My AONE fellowship project was getting an alcohol withdrawal program up and running on my ninth-floor unit. I had very mixed emotions trying to make this decision, as I did not want to give up either of my units, after the last 4 years of time and dedication to the staff.

"After many conversations with my husband, director, and assistant managers, I decided to take both units on the fourth floor to make myself more accessible to the staff. I really had to think about them and not about me. My fourth-floor unit had opportunities for improvement from our staff engagement survey that were in direct relation to my availability to them. Because I was between two units on different floors, it was harder for me to be visible. I knew that they truly needed me more on the fourth floor. Additionally, with the support of my amazing other nurse manager colleagues, we are managing all the units as a service line team. I could not do this without them. I have inherited an amazing group of staff on 4–6 unit that are happy to be staying open and to have some consistency in management.

"My assistant manager chose to stay on the ninth floor to carry on the alcohol program, since she also had invested so much time with it. The good news is, back in April, I was able to expand some of the services of the alcohol program to the eight other medicine units we have here, so I will still run the project and hopefully see it through hospital-wide.

"Moving forward, I know that what is going to make me successful is riding the wave of the change and being flexible. I have already had meet and greets with the staff on the new unit and am asking them three very specific questions. What do you love about 4–6? What do you want to change about 4–6? And what tools and equipment do you need on 4–6? The staff seem receptive thus far and I hope they are happy to see that I am listening to them and making the changes they want and not changing the things they love about the unit.

"This was a tactic I used in the past when I had to open from scratch my 4–7. We opened in 2010, and I had to gain the trust and respect from the staff by including them in the decision making on the unit. I am a part of their team, here working for them, and being their voice."

Deirdre D.
Manager, General Medicine

◇◇◇◇◇◇◇◇◇◇

"When I first came into the role as director of our department, I had been made aware of huge dissatisfaction among our nursing staff related to scheduling. Many had already left or planned to leave. One of my first priorities was to assemble a cross-sectional team of nurses from our unit who could begin to work together with me to find solutions. We agreed up front on several key points:

- The group was given decision-making authority.
- Regardless of the outcome, the group agreed that everyone would need to agree that they could "live with the outcome."
- The primary challenges were identified and prioritized.
- A time frame for the work was clearly defined. We agreed to meet six times, for 2 hours each time, over 2 months.
- As the director, I would facilitate, provide input when information I had could have an impact on a decision that was being considered, and provide background.
- The team would have time to discuss, come to resolution and decide on a course of action.
- At the conclusion of the task force/ad hoc committee, the decisions would become scheduling guidelines and distributed to the department for implementation at the beginning of the fiscal year.

"The outcome of this task force was amazing. The group came together and discussed some incredibly hot topics, they felt heard, and resolved together. In the end, they created guidelines addressing seniority, holidays, PTO, schedule requests, weekend makeup, shared governance involvement, and several other related items. These outcomes became guidelines that were distributed and implemented as promised. The staff were surveyed a year later and asked how satisfied they were with scheduling compared to a year earlier. The results were incredibly satisfying to this team. Prior to the task force, only 25% of the nurses were satisfied or highly satisfied with scheduling. A year after the implementation, 75% of the nurses indicated that they were satisfied or highly satisfied with scheduling.

"As a continuation, this team took this work further by being the first unit to do more with scheduling. They led the organization in scheduling practices by implementing self-scheduling using Kronos because they had already been successful in building positive scheduling process. Later, recognized as a needed practice, the organization developed a scheduling policy based on the foundational work of this unit that is now implemented organization wide, and is now in the process of implementing self-scheduling through Kronos on all in-patient units, using this unit as a platform.

"I truly believe the action that led to success is setting expectations, creating a culture of buy-in from the beginning, bringing the right people to the table, deferring to expertise (we brought in our scheduler for all meetings), listening more than you talk as a leader, and communicating the rationale and outcomes. The attitudes that lead to success are openness, approachability, listening for influence, willingness to change, and taking risk. This was one of the most successful and enjoyable experiences for all of us and created great relationships along the way."

Lori P.

Clinical Director, Nursing Specialty Resource Unit

◇◇◇◇◇◇◇◇◇◇◇

"I work in an intensive care unit, which has restricted visitation. About a year ago we made a decision to allow patients to have up to four people at the bedside. This was a decision made after a lot of thought and discussion. Previously, we had only allowed three people in the room at one time. This created great angst among families because the family was frequently forced to make tough decisions on who to bring back. Examples include blended families with two step-parents—which step-parent gets to be back at the bedside? How often do they switch out, etc.? Another example is with grandparents—who do you decide to bring back first, grandma or grandpa? If the patient is critically ill, who helps support this third person—do you expect the grieving parents to help the grandparent through this?

"Adding a fourth person allowed an additional support person for these difficult situations and took away many of these difficult decisions. However, when we made this decision, the staff were up in arms! They felt we had made the decision 'willy nilly' and neglected to consider what the repercussions would be for staff. They were certain this would create issues—especially from a crowd control standpoint—and would only add to our already intense visitation issues.

"A year later, I'm happy to report the staff griping lasted briefly, but the benefits can still be felt today. The number of complaints is down from both staff and families and this has freed up a significant amount of time for managers and charge RNs to focus on other duties and responsibilities.

"*Why was it a success and what did I say or do?* Ultimately, I shared our logic behind expanding visitation and told staff we would 'trial' the change. I let them know that we would be tracking issues that arose, and if the cons began to outweigh the pros, that we would change back. I think knowing that we would track issues and that the change wasn't 'set in stone' helped ease some of the angst. The irony behind it all is that there was never a single issue raised. The staff got worked up and anxious about hypothetical situations that never came to fruition. I had been in my role 3 to 4 years and dealt with visitation issues on almost a daily basis. I wanted to implement this change years earlier, but when I vetted it through a few staff or managers I received a lot of push back. When I finally followed my gut and did what I felt was the right thing to do, it worked out and I wished I had done it sooner!"

Erik M. Clinical Director, Pediatric Intensive Care Unit

◇◇◇◇◇◇◇◇◇◇◇

"We are really going through lots of changes right now in the women, infants, and children department. We are renovating multiple areas, having new monitors installed in our NICU, changing our focus in newborn nursery to a mother/baby practice, and moving our transition nursery to decentralized areas. It can feel overwhelming to leaders and staff alike.

"What seems to be most helpful is making regular rounds with the nurses and support staff to make sure everyone has a good idea of what is being done and the work that is scheduled. Gathering the feedback of the nurses and support staff alike has been instrumental in making sure we have planned for the most important aspects of care through these changes. A lot of the day is spent just being out on the unit and talking with staff about their ideas and making sure they feel calm about the plans, while being able to bring forth the concerns they have to key leaders. This can be fun when you are able to make some positive changes based on the feedback received.

"Another aspect that is difficult is when we have had to move offices and placement of various support alignment services. What seems to help us make these moves more readily is to keep the patient in mind, with the common goal for what will support the patient best. If we focus our efforts in this way as we are making the changes, it helps us to make better decisions and to forge through any difficulties.

"The change can be challenging, and it is rewarding when you begin to see positive outcomes for patients!"

Debbie B.
Manager, Neonatal Nurseries

◇◇◇◇◇◇◇◇◇◇◇

"We've all seen change. Whether it's new leadership, equipment, processes, whatever the case may be, change happens. As leaders in nursing, we continually adapt and promote change in the best way possible to have the most minimal negative affect. So with this, I'm choosing to speak about personal change. Change that started with a phone call from my CNO in 2012 asking me to apply for the nurse manager fellowship. Over the course of 2013, the nurse manager fellowship was the spark!

It completely lit my fire to desire more, achieve more, and perfect more. Because of this spark, I'm more engaged at work. My goals are set higher than ever before and I'm confident my change in the outlook of leadership will and has positively affected my staff, departments, and hospital. This spark gave me a drive for higher education and I'm happy to say I started my MSN program. The nurse manager fellowship was the spark for my biggest change."

Morgan T.
Nurse Manager, Clinical Transition Unit

◇◇◇◇◇◇◇◇◇◇

"[We had a] successful closure of a general medical unit last year. Our team worked very hard the prior year to make improvements in CAUTI rates and use of a Foley catheter removal protocol; decrease our fall rates (we went over 100 days without a fall, a hospital record at the time); and improve our HCAHP scores (one month, we exceeded our goals in eight out of eight domains). Staff morale was high, patients were happy, and physicians noticed the positive changes.

"The hospital administration opted to close the unit, and dispense the staff to other units with vacancies. While this was very upsetting news, the staff transitioned very well. I believe the support, encouragement, and rewards from the above initiatives helped build our team, provided nurses with a sense of working to the fullest extent of their licensure. In turn, the positive outcomes we achieved made our nurses very desirable to other nursing units.

"I continue to see many of the nurses in their new roles. They have blossomed, learned new skills, and are welcomed by their new teams. Additionally, several nurses now work in our Visiting Nurses of Schenectady, where leadership is pleased to have these wonderful nurses in their new roles."

Kathleen G.
Manager, Case Management and Social Work

Your Thoughts?

Pick one or more of these examples of peer wisdom about change to explore.
What lessons from your own experiences come to mind as you read these stories?

....

....

....

....

....

....

Q & Q: Quote and Question

Consider each quote about motivation and answer the follow-up question in light of your experiences.

> Q: We can't be afraid of change. You may feel very secure in the pond that you are in, but if you never venture out of it, you will never know that there is such a thing as an ocean, a sea.
>
> C. JoyBell C.

Q: **Describe a time when you ventured out of your pond.**

....

....

....

....

> Q: "Those who cannot change their mind, cannot change anything."
>
> **George Bernard Shaw**

Q: **Describe situation that required that you to change your mind.**

....

....

....

....

> Q: "The trouble with the future is that it is not what it used to be."
>
> **Yogi Berra**

Q: **How does this statement explain why you—and members of your team—resist change?**

....

....

Q: "Some people change when they see light; others when they feel the heat."

Carla Schroeder

Q: **Describe a recent change or innovation you have been trying to introduce. Who are the members of your team who saw the light and who felt the heat? How might you coach those who waited for the heat to see the light?**

Q: "I am always doing that which I cannot do, in order that I may learn how to do it."

Pablo Picasso

Q: **Describe a time you did something you could not do and learned to do it. What was the outcome?**

Q: "In the end, change sticks when it becomes the way we do this around here."

John Kotter

Q: **Describe an example in your leadership practice that demonstrates this idea.**

Deep Dive Resources: Change Leadership

Books

Cooperrider, D., Whitney, D., & Stavros, J. (2008). *Appreciative inquiry handbook for leaders of change.* Berrett Koehler.

Duhigg, C. (2012). *The power of habit: Why we do what we do in business and in life.* Random House.

Dyer, J., Gregerson, H., & Christensen, C. (2011). *The innovator's DNA.* Harvard Business Review Press.

Heath, C., & Heath, D. (2010). *Switch: How to change when change is hard.* Crown Business.

Hickey, M. & Beck-Kritek, P. (2012). *Change leadership in nursing: How change occurs in a complex hospital system.* Springer.

Kegan, R., & Laskow-Leahy, L. (2009). *Immunity to change.* Harvard Business Review Press.

Kotter, J., & Cohen, D. (2012). *The heart of change.* Harvard Business Review.

Malloch, K., & Porter-O'Grady, T. (2008). *The quantum leader: Applications for the new world of work.* Jones and Bartlett.

May, N., & Becker, D. (2011). *Appreciative inquiry in healthcare.* Crown Custom.

McKergow, M., & Clarke, J. (2007). *Solutions focus working: 80 real life lessons for successful organizational change.* Solutions Books.

Musselwhite, C. (2010). *Dangerous opportunity: Making change work.* Discovery Learning.

Pascale, R., Sternin, J., & Sternin, M. (2010). *The power of positive deviance: How unlikely innovators solve the world's toughest problems.* Harvard Business Press.

Sare, M., & Ogilvie, L. (2010). *Strategic planning for nurses: Change management in healthcare.* Jones and Bartlett.

Professional Journals

Bowers, N. (2011). Managing change by empowering staff. *Nursing Times, 107*(32/33), 19–21.

Lehman, K. L. (2008). Change management: Magic or mayhem? *Journal for Nurses in Staff Development, 24*(4), 176–184.

MacPhee, M. (2007). Strategies and tools for managing change. *The Journal of Nursing Administration, 37*(9), 405–413.

Morjikian, R. L., Kimball, B., & Joynt, J. (2007). Leading change: The nurse executive's role in implementing new care delivery models. *The Journal of Nursing Administration, 37*(9), 399–404.

Richer, M. C., Ritchie, J., & Marchionni, C. (2009). If we can't do more, let's do it differently! Using appreciative inquiry to promote innovative ideas for better health care work environments. *Journal of Nursing Management, 17*(8), 947–955.

Salmela, A., Eriksson, K., & Fagerstrom, L. (2012). Leading change: A three-dimensional model of nurse leaders' main tasks and roles during a change process. *Journal of Advanced Nursing, 68*(2), 423–433.

Skelton-Green, J., Simpson, B., & Scott, J. (2007). An integrated approach to change leadership. *Nursing Leadership, 20*(3), 399–404.

Trajkovski, S., Schmied, V., Vickers, M., & Jackson, D. (2013). Using appreciative inquiry to transform health care. *Contemporary Nurse 45*(1), 95–100.

Videos

Kotter, J. *The heart of change* [Video]. YouTube. https://www.youtube.com/watch?v=1NKti9MyAAw

TEDx. (2013, January). *Six keys to leading positive change: Rosabeth Moss Kanter at TEDxBeaconStreet* [Video]. YouTube. https://www.youtube.com/watch?v=owU5aTNPJbs

Figure Credits

Fig. 6.1a: Copyright © 2010 Depositphotos/colorvsbw.

Fig. 6.1b: Copyright © 2014 Depositphotos/NatalyaA.

Fig. 6.1c: Copyright © 2020 Depositphotos/mentalmind.

Fig. 6.1d: Copyright © 2017 Depositphotos/worldofvector.

Fig. 6.1e: Copyright © 2014 Depositphotos/yobro10.

Fig. 6.1f: Copyright © 2013 Depositphotos/interatimages.

Sisu

Responding to Adversity

"Every night, when I take the elevator up to my floor, I call upon an inner strength to get me through one more night. I became a nurse to help. I never believed it would require a special courage, but now I know that is true. It's not just me, the whole team, the whole floor; the whole hospital is calling upon a unique type of fortitude that allows us to get the job done."

◇◇◇◇◇◇◇◇◇◇◇◇◇◇◇◇◇◇

In the first spring of the COVID-19 pandemic, I received a gallant and gutsy email from Erin D., an ICU nurse at Lenox Hill Hospital in New York. Her words reminded me that every nurse engages in acts of leadership: Every nurse leads a team of one.

She describes how this "horrifying disease has allowed me to witness acts of love on a scale I would not have imagined." She recalls a loving, long-married couple—each with a deadly prognosis—in beds on separate floors. She ferried the wife in a wheelchair to her husband's side so that they could die together. By the time Erin returned to her station, the wife's bed had been assigned to another patient.

"No time to be sad," Erin said. "I had another patient to care for. As nurses, we have all developed the ability to compartmentalize illness and death, but not at this extreme, unprecedented level. *We are drawing upon a heretofore untouched well of strength and determination.* There is no end in sight. I am sure we will continue to be tested above and beyond. But I know we will do it and we will do it together."

The Finnish language has a word for Erin's fortitude, inventiveness, and untouched well of strength: *sisu* (pronounced see-soo). Emilia Elisabet Lahti, the first researcher to a conduct a systematic study of sisu, defined it as the extraordinary courage and determination that surfaces *only* in response to adversity, suffering, frustration, and hardship.[1] It is almost like a spare tank of gas, Lahti explains; its benefits are because of adversity, not in spite of it.

In this final laboratory—with a slightly altered format—I will highlight stories from frontline nurses and nurse leaders, drawn from my sisu research at Lenox Hill Hospital to create a podcast during the first spring of the COVID-19 pandemic.[2] Other exemplars of sisu will also include more recent reports from nurse leaders.

These exemplars will illustrate three key elements of sisu gleaned from Emilia Elisabet Lahti's groundbreaking studies, and include my communications with Lahti. Keep your lived experiences of sisu in mind. These elements will provide a springboard for you to examine and experiment with a series of micro actions and cognitive strategies associated with sisu.

The Study of Sisu

The word is 500 years old. Etymologically, "sisu" comes from a Finnish root word that implies "inner" or "inside." This is one reason it is sometimes translated as "guts" or "inner strength." It reemerged in Finland's vocabulary, inspired by the perseverance of Finnish soldiers who fought in the punishing cold of the 1939 Winter War.[3] Outnumbered by the powerful forces of the Soviet army's invasion, the Finns persisted with guerilla tactics (like wearing white as camouflage in the snow) and preserved Finland's independence.

Since then, sisu, as a hidden source of reserved power, has become a key element in Finnish culture. To wit: If you want to insult a Finn, tell them that they lack sisu! Yet it is believed to be relevant beyond the Finnish shores. The shiny idea here is that, in each of us, there is more strength than meets the eye.

I discovered the psychological construct of sisu when I worked on a Fulbright grant with nurse leaders at Helsinki University Hospital. Here, I encountered the work of researcher Emilia Elisabet Lahti, Finland's foremost authority on sisu. Lahti analyzed more than 1,000 responses from Finns and others knowledgeable about sisu. Her article, "Embodied Fortitude: An Introduction to the Finnish Concept of Sisu," as well as her international public platform, have carried this concept into the world outside her country.[4] Lahti speaks of sisu as "a fire that does not fade—no matter what. It is a power that springs from deep within—allowing you to try one more time."

Sisu is not macho John Wayne grit or the legendary mental toughness of Serena Williams. Lahti considers it to be the next gear beyond fortitude. It begins where grit and perseverance end—a deeper reserve of power within all of us.

At this writing, empirical studies like Lahti's are in their infancy. Current research includes efforts to quantify and measure sisu, to compare it to other dimensions of hardiness and resilience and to validate it as a psychological construct outside of the cultural context of Finland.[5, 6]

The most promising studies are being conducted by psychologist Ilmari Närväinen at the University of Helsinki and research scientist Johanna Närväinen at VTT Technical Research Center of Finland. They are mapping beneficial and harmful sisu, with questionnaires, labs tests, and physiologic measurement. With Lahti, they created a sisu scale and found associations between sisu and well-being.[7]

For our purposes, we can return to Erin D.'s example to illustrate Lahti's seminal descriptions of sisu's three key elements.

- *Sisu is extraordinary perseverance that allows us to move beyond a prior view of our mental and physical capacities.* So we finish what we start, despite the difficulty, and choose integrity over shortcuts.

  This element is captured in Erin's description of "special courage" and "calling upon a unique kind of fortitude that allows us to get the job done."

- *Sisu allows us to draw upon previously hidden, untapped sources of power and strength.* When faced with a challenge, we access a reserve of energy (one that we didn't know we had). We experience a second wind. This element is expressed when Erin suggests, "We are drawing upon a heretofore untouched well of strength and determination."

- *Sisu is also an action mindset that allows us to face up to fears and take action in moments of suffering and challenge.* We envision a story where we can succeed, create bridges across barriers, and unleash creativity in daunting circumstances. Erin describes the essence of her action mindset. "There is no end in sight. I am sure we will continue to be tested above and beyond. But I know we will do it and we will do it together."

Element	Attributes
Key #1 Sisu is extraordinary perseverance.	~You go beyond your previous view of your mental or physical capacities. ~You finish what you start—despite the difficulty. ~You do what seemed impossible. ~You show integrity and do not take shortcuts at the expense of quality.
Key #2 Sisu is a latent source of reserved—but not yet presented—energy and power.	~You are able to gain access to a power and energy reserve (one that you did not know you had) during great challenge. ~You move toward a vision of where you might go if you dare to try. ~You get a second wind. ~Your energy and resolve seem to appear, as if summoned by adversity.
Key #3 Sisu is an action mindset.	~You take action against slim odds. ~You show a courageous and hopeful attitude toward challenges. ~You are able to imagine a story where you succeed. ~You face up to your fears. ~You transform a barrier into a bridge to action. ~You are creative as a result of hardship or frustration.

These three elements are also present in the words of Emily F., who described working five 13-hour shifts in a row. She details her extraordinary perseverance. "I am both completely physically exhausted and mentally drained. I could probably sit here and complain about how my feet are swollen and throbbing, how I have a headache from the tight mask, how

I have cried three times today already, or how I miss my family. But, I am choosing not to. And this is why: Today I had the honor and privilege to 'send off' a Navy veteran—to give him the good-bye that he deserved."

She gains access to an inner energy reserve. "It was at this moment I had to call on my inner strength and courage. It no longer mattered that I was exhausted, that I had not eaten lunch, that I had charting to do. All that mattered was this patient and his family. They were my strength, my courage. If they could be strong is this moment, so could I."

Emily described her team's action mindset: transforming a barrier into a poignant bridge by jumping into action. "We called the family in, gathered hospital workers who were veterans, got the music ready. We all gowned up; the family said their good-byes. We played the Star-Spangled Banner and we all gave him his final salute. He passed away shortly after. It was beautiful and it is this moment that will carry me into my next shift."

I contacted Emilia Elisabet Lahti, to share some of these soul-stirring stories and to ask her to apply her research about sisu as a lens through which to view the exceptional responses of frontline health care workers. In our lively dialogue, Lahti called sisu "the friendly darkness of adversity."[8]

She elaborated, "The sisu these nurses describe has appeared in a moment of extreme adversity; it is invoked by an experience that calls them to stretch and expand. Sisu is our ability to channel a moment and open the pathway to a latent existing strength that resides within us."

The COVID-19 pandemic is such a moment, explained Lahti. "We are witnessing a global expression of sisu. We see nurses and health care providers digging to reach layers of strength they did not know existed. They are stepping into their previously unpresented strength."

In Lahti's view, sisu can also be brought into expression in groups where a team of people becomes a united field of force in pursuit of solving a situation that seems impossible and unsolvable. Kris B. explained, "In hard times, there are two factors that motivate me. The first factor is my coworkers. Hard work is contagious; so when teamwork and the support of the people around me rally to overcome adversity, I want to elevate and show strength alongside theirs."

ICU nurse Joseph P. described his second wind, powered by the combined strength of this team. This power allowed him to move toward a vision of how the team can—and will—meet this moment. "At the beginning of the shift, I felt defeated. Like I ran out of fumes and now had to push the car from the back while no one was steering. I had just seen four patients in a row and was recovering from that and felt like there was no way I could handle three more ICU patients that were not stable. But through teamwork, camaraderie, and hard work we were able to do something special. And I absolutely couldn't have done it on my own. It's a privilege to be a nurse, now more than ever; and I am confident that our team is more than capable of seeing this through if we work together."

REFLECTION

Map your experiences in leading yourself and others with the three elements of sisu.

Describe a time when your physical and mental resources felt used up and yet *you perservered*—finished what you started and went beyond your previous views of your mental or physical capacity.

....

....

....

....

....

Describe an instance when you felt defeated by fear or failure but were able to *gain access to a power and energy reserve* you did not know you had—and to move toward a desired direction or goal.

....

....

....

....

....

Describe an experience in your leadership when you wanted to achieve something, and felt as if you faced incredibly long odds, yet you were able *to envision your success and step toward action.*

....

....

....

....

....

Consider one caveat: All sisu is not created equal. We need not valorize every struggle. Lahti warns against "stubborn sisu" or "silent relentlessness." When you access deep reserves of energy, you must also take care not to accidentally deplete them. Her study data suggests that too much sisu—and not knowing when to stop—can result in burnout, exhaustion, disconnection, and making unreasonable demands on others.

Sisu will help us take the next step, or the first one, Lahti explained. But the outcome of that action will depend on how we use it. In that sense, sisu can be constructive or destructive. We must also underline the need for replenishment, both in the moment and as a further source of sustaining your inner strength.

Joshua T. describes how to meet the moment: "It takes a lot for me to be sent 'over the edge' and when I do, it takes a lot for me to tap into my inner strength. A tactic I've learned is to take a moment for sensory deprivation. I go into the bathroom, lock the door, turn the lights off, and stand in silence. I tune my ears to listen to only my breath and I stay present for as long as I can. I do my very best to stay in that moment and carry it with me."

In our research exploring personal leadership, my colleague Gary Wenet and I detailed the way leaders recharged their batteries, reinvigorated themselves, and restored their perspective. Rather than seeking balance, exemplary leaders sought replenishment through counterpoint and contrast. One executive captured this counterpoint: "Unless you have another world your mind can exist in, you cannot be refreshed when you return to the work where you are supposed to be a leader."[9]

Since all of the resources of your leadership—whether clinical, strategic, or interpersonal—are renewable resources, the only way you can renew them is to take time off from using them. Replenishment through counterpoint requires making thoughtful choices about crafting time away from work to experience a different sense of self, purpose, and time.

REFLECTION

Compare notes with Amanda S., an executive director of a nursing organization, who describes power-washing the brick walkway of her in-laws' home. She lost track of time as she kept pointing the powerful nozzle between the bricks, splattering water and dirt everywhere. Taking a break, Amanda looked in the mirror and saw that her face and clothes were soaked and streaked with mud. "This was definitely a different view of myself!" she said. We can also note that she experienced a different sense of purpose and time.

Describe ways you express a different sense of yourself—a marked contrast to your work self in your time away from your leadership role—through friendship, politics, spirituality, family ritual, arts, athletics, or burning interests.

....

....

....

....

....

Describe ways you have experienced a different sense of purpose and satisfaction out-side of work, ones that distinctly contrast with your devoted health care leadership (e.g., power-washing instead of prioritizing budget items).

....

....

....

....

....

Your days are packed with deadlines and a sense of a job that is never done. Describe the ways you craft a different sense of time in the hours away from work.

....

....

....

....

....

In his *Treatise on Painting*, Leonardo da Vinci advises, "Leave off work and take a little relaxation. Because when you come back to it you are a better judge."[10] Da Vinci was convinced the replenishment found in time away from work was crucial to incubating and generating energy for a refreshed perspective and new ideas.

Describe a situation in which you took time to replenish your energy and came back to your leadership as "a better judge."

....

....

....

....

....

Four Cognitive Strategies for Sisu

Hold your experiences up to the light as we consider four cognitive strategies—and meaningful actions—that are associated with constructive sisu. Identify your best practices and plan to experiment with actionable strategies to enrich your resilient leadership.

Strategy	Actions	Your best practices
Discernment	~Find meaning in the midst of reality. ~Distinguish faith from facts.	
Self-efficacy	~Draw upon internal locus of control. ~Lead with a growth mindset.	
Deliberate thought	~Manage your attention. ~Envision outcomes.	
Bricolage	~Create novel solutions with existing resources. ~Initiate improvisation.	

Discernment

Discernment is a combination of sense making and reflective thinking—a vital process for leading self and others.[11, 12] It is the kind of decision making that looks at all sides of the elephant. In the realm of sisu, discernment provides a means of distinguishing faith from facts,[13] seeking meaning in confronting reality, and avoiding stubborn sisu.

The behavioral components of discernment in leadership have been spelled out by various researchers.[14, 15] Among them: willingness to accept uncertainty, kicking it with common sense, seeking new ways to look at familiar views, imagining future possibilities, emotional self-awareness, factoring hunches into decisions, paying attention to body cues or fleeting thoughts, and protecting quiet time to reflect and find meaning.

REFLECTION

How do you know when it is time to pause for replenishment or stop the struggle? Study this painting of the much-told Greek myth of Sisyphus—a former king sentenced to silent, relentless sisu: condemned by the peeved Zeus for eternity to roll a boulder up to the top a hill, only to have it roll down again.[16] Give Sisyphus another look. What comes to mind?

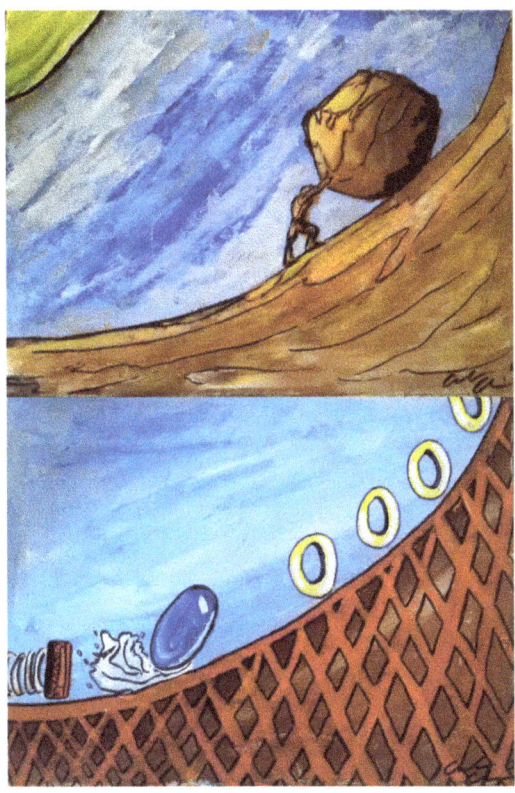

FIGURE 7.1

....

....

....

....

....

....

....

REFLECTION

In his book, *The Myth of Sisyphus*, Albert Camus casts Sisyphus as a stand-in for our struggles against the absurdity of life.[17] He focuses on what Sisyphus is thinking as the rock rolls down the hill.

Camus wonders if Sisyphus might choose find joy rather than despair in his rolling stone. He even suggests, "The struggle itself would be enough to fill our hearts." Do you agree? Describe a challenging experience, a struggle that shaped your point of view.

....

....

....

....

....

EXPERIMENT

The reality testing of discernment poses two crucial questions—and you must ask both. First, am I going to pack in it now, after everything I have been through to get to this point? Just as important: Is this goal achievable; can this challenge be met? In other words: Is this a workable situation or is this my wishful thinking?

Self-Efficacy

Sisu, an action mindset, is a sibling to the well-studied leadership practice of self-efficacy.[18] Confidence and self-efficacy, two concepts grounded by a positive belief in self, and often used interchangeably, are widely considered to be fundamental building blocks of leadership.[19, 20] Self-efficacy, as first defined by Albert Bandura, is powered by the confident belief in our capabilities to organize and complete actions to produce a given outcome.[21]

Confident self-efficacy and a sense of agency embolden acts of sisu. An essential component of self-efficacy resides in what psychologist Julian Rotter called locus of control.[22] He contrasts two modes of thinking—each one will have an effect on the capacity to act with sisu.

Sisu will be difficult for leaders who approach challenges with what Rotter describes as an *external locus of control*. They believe that outcomes are largely beyond their control and are determined more by powerful others, luck, fate, or chance. With this mental stance, leaders and team members are more likely to give up or give in to circling the drain of emotions and are less likely to try to influence others, because they don't think they will succeed. Their defeating thought bubbles: *"What's the point? This is impossible. No one will listen to me."*

Rotter contrasts this approach with an *internal locus of control*, a perspective that allows for leaders to be emboldened actors—to draw upon sisu—in meeting challenges. Leaders with an internal locus of control believe that outcomes are the result of their own behavior, decisions, and hard work.

They are less likely to give up or give in to Debbie Downer emotions and more likely to attempt to influence other people, because they believe that their efforts will be successful. They wonder: "What might work?" "What if I tried … ?" "How can I convince my team to … ?"

EXPERIMENT

Choose one of two statements in Rotter's locus of control scale. (A link to the full test can be found in the Deep Dive Resources.) How might your choice influence your capacity to act with sisu in a challenging or adverse situation?

....
....
....
....
....

a. "I have often found that what is going to happen will happen."

....
....
....
....
....

b. "Trusting to fate has never turned out as well for me as making a decision to take a definite course of action."

....

....

....

....

....

Rose May C. reveals sisu as an action mindset that allows her to face her fears, extend herself in moments of suffering, and take action in the most daunting circumstances—even with no guarantee of success. She sees herself as an agent with an internal control of the situation. This is the essence of self-efficacy expressed in moments of sisu. In Rose May's story, it is also an example of what leadership educator John Maxwell calls "failing forward":[23] "Today was my first day at work really dealing with a COVID unit. I was not ready!! It felt like the zombie apocalypse. At times it feels as if I am at war, even though last I checked, I am a civilian. Today it is hard to picture the light at the end of the tunnel."

But then, she summoned her sisu and addressed the virus directly: "That's OK, Corona, I was not ready today. But tomorrow is another day. Scoreboard: CORONA: 1 ME: 0. I'm made of tougher stuff than you. Corona, you won't get me again. Enjoy your win; I'm in it in for the long haul. I will dig deep, deeper than I ever needed to. I will do it for my family, your family, my brothers and sisters at the frontline, for me, for humanity."

Psychologist Carol Dweck's research gives us a front-row seat to consider Rose May's effortful sisu.[24] Her research introduced the idea that a growth mindset—as contrasted with a fixed mindset—drives self-efficacy and agency. In sum: A fixed mindset is the belief that your strengths and capacities are static. A growth mindset is the belief that challenge is a bridge to growth and that your effort and persistence can provide a path to mastery. Clearly, a growth mindset contributes to self-efficacy.

We see that, at first, Rose May admits, "I was not ready today." But if she had believed that her capacity to meet this challenge was fixed or limited, she would have felt defeated. Instead she says, "OK, Corona. I was not ready today, but tomorrow is another day. You won't get me again." Here she taps into the growth mindset where her abilities are not static and she can believe that her efforts will carry her forward.

REFLECTION

After her initial sense of being overwhelmed, Rose May lost her fear of trying. Describe an exceptionally challenging situation where you drew upon sisu to power your sense of agency. Did you have to overcome a fixed mindset to embrace a growth mindset? What were your effortful actions?

....

....

....

....

....

REFLECTION

Describe a time when you encouraged sisu and honored the effort of your team without denying the difficulty or adversity they faced.

....

....

....

....

....

Deliberate Thought

It is instructive to view sisu in the light of decades of research about self-leadership.[25] Management psychologists Charles Neck and Christopher Manz have underlined the electric dynamic between thoughts and behavior.[26, 27] With this understanding, it is possible to unpack several ways in which sisu—an action mindset—is the result of deliberate thought patterns.

The influence of our inner narratives (name-checked in the popular press as "self-talk") on our actions has been explored in a number of intriguing studies in the fields of sports, counseling psychology, education, and leadership. For example, organizational psychologists

Steven Rogelberg and Logan Justice found that constructive inner narrative was a stopgap against work stress and linked to leaders' mastery and creativity.[28]

A 30-item self-leadership scale includes three now-familiar aspects of sisu: self-cueing, positive inner narrative, and visualization of successful performance. Each of these demands a deliberate thought process.[29]

Consider the story of Mike J., now a CNO, looking back on his feelings of exhaustion in the months after Hurricane Sandy. Many other Manhattan hospitals remained closed, requiring his team to take on more and more patients. He drew upon his sisu by maintaining a line of sight to purpose, with deliberate thoughts that focus on patient care. This framing of the situation influences his capacity to meet the challenge.

As Mike explains, "That first night of the hurricane it was hard to find the strength or energy to move even one more patient from the waiting room into a treatment area. All hands were on deck in the beginning. We had to intake dozens of patients from hospitals that were being evacuated in the middle of the night. But that night isn't when I, or anyone else, ran out of energy. It was in the months that followed. I think each person reached their low at various times in those subsequent months."

He describes the expression of his sisu: "Only those of us who lived the surge from the beginning knew what it used to be like versus what we were facing now, weeks after the hurricane waters had receded. It was with this knowledge that I was able to dig down even deeper, knowing that it wasn't that patient in the waiting room that was causing this low-low, it was all the days before compounded onto this one. But, I had the power to help that patient, so that is what I did. Then the next one, then the next one. And eventually, things got back to normal."

Mike's inner dialogue, connecting his line of sight to the care of patients, was his inner cue for meeting the situation with sisu.[30] When Mike detailed "digging down even deeper" he displayed his ability to manage his attention in line with his mission.[31]

 REFLECTION

Describe a situation of challenge or adversity when you demonstrated sisu by maintaining line of sight to your commitment to your team and the health of your patients.

....

....

....

....

....

Social psychologist Karl Weick would dub Mike's deliberate thoughts *future perfect thinking*.[32] His inner narrative guided him to imagine his "power to help the patient and the next one and the next." More poetically, Emilia Elisabet Lahti evokes the brilliance of dreaming: Mike created a vision of himself in the future—one where he meets the challenge and moves beyond it.[33]

EXPERIMENT

Go back to the future. David Cooperrider's approach of appreciative inquiry has also drawn us to dreaming and its effect on desired outcomes. He encourages us to meet challenges by using sparky questions to envision what might be.[34]

As a practical matter, this means that when you or your team are stressed and scorched by current situations, you might ask, What will I/we be doing when this is no longer a problem? Can I/we think about 1 year from now—with the challenge or hardship in our rearview mirror? What steps will I/we need to take to make this possible?

REFLECTION

Pose the miracle question. Ask yourself/your team to imagine this: A miracle happened while you were reading this chapter. The clear and present challenge or obstacle you are facing today is moving toward a promising outcome.

Describe the first thing you would notice. What is one small change that might have made this possible? What other actions could have contributed to forward movement?

....

....

....

....

....

Bricolage

Leaders who are creative as a result of challenge or adversity practice the cognitive and actionable strategy of bricolage—resolving problems with resources at hand. The word is derived from the French verb *bricoleur* ("to tinker"). It was introduced by anthropologist

Claude Lévi-Strauss, who was intrigued with the way societies create novel solutions by using resources that already exist.[35]

Later research refers to bricolage as the creation of something new from little available resources, or by combining various limited resources.[36] Here bricolage is characterized as a kind of practical intelligence and inventiveness that moves you to the next point. We saw this in Emily F.'s creating an end-of-life ceremony for a Marine veteran and his family. (She gathered veterans on her staff and found patriotic music on her phone.)

Television's pop culture icon of bricolage, MacGyver (and MacGruber, his satiric stand-in on *Saturday Night Live*) demonstrated outsized sisu by creating solutions with what was immediately available, say, bubble gum or a paper clip.

In a more scholarly depiction, researcher Mary Gobbi writes about nursing practice as embodied bricolage.[37] She details practitioners drawing on the "shards and fragments" of the situation at hand to resolve the needs of individual patients in their care.

Tuyen K. is an exemplar of the bricolage that Gobbi has evoked. She describes meeting the needs of a Buddhist family whose father had died. Note the ways Tuyen locates available resources—literally gathering shards and fragments:[38]

"I asked them repeatedly about calling a funeral home; about making arrangements. They did not answer my questions. I finally asked, 'What do you need us to do?' The daughter told me the family believed that his death was another journey. They wanted to perform a ritual to prepare him: to put a little gold and rice underneath his tongue."

Tuyen jumped into action. "I thought, where can we get the gold? One of his daughters said, 'I can go home and scrape it off one of my rings.' We sent her home in a cab. The kitchen was closed, but we needed some rice. I asked a team member to go to the kitchen to see what he could do. He got two steps away and asked, 'How much?' and 'Does it need to be cooked?' Each time, another daughter answered our questions. When he came back with a bowl of uncooked rice and the other daughter returned, they placed one grain of rice and a small scraping of gold in their father's mouth. And we were able to fulfill their requests."

 REFLECTION

Describe a time when (like Tuyen) you or your team drew upon "shards and fragments" of a situation to meet a challenge.

....

....

....

....

....

Rather than waiting for turbulent times to inspire bricolage, train your team to imagine through improvisation. Jazz musicians improvise solos with the same chord progression, comedians riff on the same joke. In a similar way, you can create discussions where your team practices building on each other's ideas. Kat Koppett, a pioneer in applied improvisation, evokes the elements of bricolage. "[When you improvise] you have what you have—and what are you going to do with it?"[39]

The motivating mantra of improvisation is the phrase "yes, and."[40] This is referred to as "accepting the offer." You affirm what another person offers and build on it. In this framework, "yes, but" is considered a shut-up ploy—the enemy of creative problem solving.

EXPERIMENT

Koppett outlines a practice session: Ask for five volunteers. Pick an imaginary issue for your team (e.g., planning a spring picnic).

In round one, each person contributes one idea, and the person next to them says "yes, but"—explaining why it won't work. Every subsequent person must also say, "yes, but." Each person shuts down the previous idea.

- "Let's have the picnic at the beach."
- "Yes, but … that's too far way."
- "Yes, but … we could carpool."
- "Yes but … gas is so expensive."

In round two, each person contributes an idea and every subsequent person builds on the idea with the expression "yes, and."

- "Let's have the picnic at the beach."
- "Yes, and … we can build a campfire."
- "Yes, and … we can roast hot dogs."
- "Yes, and … we could make s'mores."

Debrief and discuss.

EXPERIMENT

Lévi-Strauss considered bricolage as a mindset where the first step is retrospective.[41] When faced with challenge or running out of steam, take step back and analyze your available resources. Then take a moment (alone or with your team) to recall past experiences that might provide clues about your present challenge.

Parting Thoughts

We close this laboratory and our work together with a stirring story from Megan H., a nurse leader who recalled her experience of sisu as a clinical nurse:

> "In the doing, our reserves feel infinite. While working directly with patients and within a clinical team, energies seem to reignite and spill into each other. I was never tired during a code. I might be gasping and feel sweat moving under my scrubs but I would push out the next compression harder and faster just as my team member advised. I never made it to my water bottle or the bathroom if a respiratory rate was 30 and not until my full 12 hours passed. But my body would feel fine and would continue to move and get everything done.
>
> "Until one morning, it didn't. I was tired and all I could see was one man's face and so many bodies. It was hard to raise my eyes and could feel my legs moving against the scrub fabric. I was spent and already applying for other jobs but still had shifts to work and a team to lead.
>
> "Instead of seeing what had passed my own eyes in the last 10 years, I looked to our team. So many looked as tired as I felt, but were moving faster than I could understand and smiling while caring for others. They each held responsibilities that no outsider could understand or ever accept. I was so proud to be part of them and felt a spark of joy and realization of community.
>
> "Almost instantly, my head raised and saw the next patient arrive and my words and motion combined and I was in sync with the stretcher and aware of every sound and need. I was still part of this team and this community filled and fueled each other."

Megan captures the essence of sisu and the brave path of learning to lead.

Ask a Nurse Leader: Peer Wise Ideas About Sisu

Pick one or more of these examples of peer wisdom to explore.
What lessons from your own experience come to mind as you read these stories?

◇◇◇◇◇◇◇◇◇◇◇

"It was a fine fall Monday morning at the hospital, as all my ICU RNs are getting ready to celebrate Thanksgiving. Around 11 a.m., I received a call from my ICU charge RN that a new cardiac arrest case is en route to ICU and we need to implement the new targeted temperature management protocol for cardiac arrest. Charge RN also mentioned that the patient is a female and in her 40s. As I entered the ICU, the patient was just wheeled in. I saw a beautiful young female, intubated, brought in by multiple ED and ICU professionals. I immediately noticed that her lipstick was still intact, which was reddish cherry color. Soon to realize that she was an elementary school teacher from one of our local schools. Also learned that she collapsed in front of her class, and by the time the EMTs arrived almost 15 minutes had passed. One of the RNs in the ICU soon recognized the patient as her daughter's first-grade teacher and started panicking, thinking that her daughter must have seen the teacher collapsing.

"As soon as the patient was stabilized in the ICU bed, I met with her parents—father a retired anesthesiologist, mother a pediatrician. The patient was declared as braindead. The ICU nursing director and I were able to accommodate all the requests of the family in preparing the room for them to stay with their daughter. We had extensive conversations with the family along with ICU providers and the hospital ethics consult, which was a very overwhelming experience. As per her driver's license information, she was a registered organ donor and conversations regarding potential organ donations were ongoing. It was a very hard decision for the family, and I was deeply involved in this case. I felt as though my heart was heavy, as whenever I entered the room, the mother would cling to me and start crying.

"As an ICU nurse educator for the past 8 years, I have had many examples of patients' untimely death, and interactions with many family members, but this case was a totally different experience. The next morning, I spent most of my time in the ICU, tried to help the parents in all the ways possible. I felt like there was nothing more we were able to provide. At this time, I thought about my professional obligations, the ethics class I had just finished as part of my PhD program, and the responsibilities I have as an ICU educator. Finally, the parents agreed for organ procurement on Wednesday (the day before Thanksgiving).

"The mother was crying all morning, she hugged me several times, I felt exhausted, but I continued to say prayers to Mother Mary to keep my inner strength and not to cry in front of them. I could see that many of my ICU RNs had tears as they continued their routine work. Although my peers suggested for me to leave the ICU, I decided to stay until she was taken to the operating room for organ procurement. I helped the parents pack and stayed in the room with them until they said their final good-byes to their daughter and accompanied the patient to the OR. This patient saved the lives of six other patients. Although I was exhausted from the past 3 days, thinking of the greatest gift of life provided to six other patients, just before Thanksgiving, helped me realize the true meaning behind Thanksgiving."

Annie G.

ICU Educator

◇◇◇◇◇◇◇◇◇◇

"As a new nurse manager, I transitioned to a new department and worked with a new service line, providers, and staff. I found myself overwhelmed and often wondering if I had made the right move. One situation that stands out as a time I had to draw on my inner strength was when a patient was highly disruptive, verbally abusive, and extremely sick. The surgical team was not engaged or able to support the staff, and I felt I didn't have the support and resources to change the situation.

"After managing the situation with no change for over 2 weeks, I decided to escalate the situation to my director and eventually the CNO. I was so passionate about this situation that I found myself in tears when I met with others, as I felt completely blocked and unable to help the patient or staff. I eventually composed myself and worked with the attending surgeon to develop a care plan that would allow the patient to receive the care she needed while supporting the staff and decreasing the verbal abuse and stress connected with the situation. After that case, I continued to advocate for a change in the care of patients with behavioral issues. After that, I also found that the attending provider was more willing to seek out my input with other patient care situations."

Nancy W.

Nurse Manager, Med-Surg Unit

◇◇◇◇◇◇◇◇◇◇

"During my first travel nurse assignment, I was assigned patients in a 'step-down' unit. The unit had two nurses caring for 11 patients. It turns out that these weren't step-down patients, but vented, unstable patients. My assignment was spread across the floor and we had no ancillary support. It was literally myself and one additional RN. The stress of that situation pushed me over the edge right away. Regardless of my opinions of how the staffing looked, at this point, I was responsible for these patients and I was there to support their needs. It takes a lot for me to be sent 'over the edge,' and when I do, it takes a lot for me to tap into my inner strength. A tactic I've learned is to take a moment for sensory deprivation. I go into the bathroom, lock the door, turn the lights off, and stand in silence. I tune my ears to listen to only my breath and I stay present for as long as I can. I do my very best to stay in that moment and carry it with me.

"As a nurse leader, I feel a little bit of that on a daily basis. It feels as if you are required to meet everyone's needs, both above and below. Even with the understanding that you can't please everyone, the expectation is that you please everyone and keep them satisfied. I can recall a time, as a new nurse leader, that I took over a department that had been without leadership for some time. The culture had been destroyed by gossip and distrust. The first staff meeting I held was a total disaster. I opened it up as a space to share concerns and it quickly became a 'B-Session.' It took every bit of restraint and insight I had to contain my words and reactions. In this situation, I tapped into my inner strength by listening to the words versus listening to the complaint. I disconnected all of the drama from the story being told and reflected on the human behavior. It softened my heart and created space for me to be present. You have to really understand people and yourself to tackle these moments."

Joshua T.
Nurse Manager

◇◇◇◇◇◇◇◇◇◇◇

"I was getting ready for work and decided to play gospel music prior to leaving the house. We were weeks into to the pandemic and listening to the words of the song, I cried for the first time. I cried because I was scared for my family, my friends, my patients, my community of healthcare workers and myself. I was scared because I did not have the answer to what this is or when this will be over. I was scared because we are all risking our lives to preserve the lives of others.

"Then, I began to listen to the words of the song. The song was telling me that God did not create me to worry, and God did not create me to fear. At that moment, I was reminded that he would take care of us. My faith took over my fear and I was able to go to work confident that I would be able to provide the support that my team needed."

Lisa P.
Director Magnet Certification

◇◇◇◇◇◇◇◇◇◇◇

"One of the departments I oversee is an outpatient infusion center which staffs four to five full-time infusion RNs and two medical assistants. We are a clinical network site of City of Hope Comprehensive Cancer Center. This was in an instance when an 84-year-old patient had a chemo reaction and subsequently passed away in our infusion department. This happened in the early stages of the COVID-19 pandemic, and patients had to come in alone for their chemo. Prior to the pandemic, patients could have one or two visitors with them throughout their treatment. With the visitor policy modified for the pandemic, however, the nurses were doubly attentive to the patients to ensure that they were ok, tolerating the treatments well, and felt emotionally supported. Friends and family usually waited outside in their vehicle and knew the nurses would call them on their phones if there were any issues or updates on the planned treatment for the day. As one of the nurses was making his rounds on his patients in the treatment chairs, and he noticed that the patient was pale, eyes were closed, and did not appear to be breathing. He started the chemo only 10 minutes prior.

"Our standard process when a patient is having a reaction to a chemotherapy is to call a 'code chemo' via overhead page. When this code chemo is triggered, the physician on-call comes to the infusion department to assess the patient and give whatever orders are necessary to relieve or reverse the reaction. Our code chemo response team is composed of infusion RNs, medical assistants, and a pharmacist, and each know their role and what standard interventions are required. As the nurse manager, I also attend all the code chemos and see where I can offer support to the staff and patient.

"As the staff initiated the code, I could see that the patient was very pale and remained unresponsive. As with any code, time seems to speed up and slow down simultaneously. The physician already asked for EMS to be dispatched and I remember the nurses taking charge and placing the patient from the infusion chair to the floor to initiate CPR. Other staff were pulling the privacy curtains, since the infusion room was at full capacity, and I was briefing the pharmacist on what happened so that she could prepare the emergency medication. I already asked one of the medical assistants to bring in the patient's daughter into our lobby so that I could meet with her and explain what was happening. I did not want to leave the nursing team prematurely since the patient remained unresponsive and the AED was going to be used. In my time as manager at the infusion department, the AED had never been used for a code and I knew the fairly young nursing team was nervous. They had never participated in a code chemo where the patient remained unresponsive beyond a few seconds. As the AED leads were being placed, the medical assistant who went to get the patient's daughter ran into the infusion room to alert us that the patient was a DNR and the daughter had the advanced directive in her purse.

"We had nothing on file to indicate the patient was DNR status, but the patient's daughter indicated that her mother recently changed her resuscitation status but had not given us a copy of the advanced directive yet. EMS was already on site at that time and had initiated CPR. The paramedic in charge spoke to the patient's daughter and updated her on the mother's status—despite CPR efforts, her mother was still unresponsive and no vital signs were detected. Given the DNR status, CPR was stopped.

"I was internally going through a rollercoaster of emotions that included, grief, fear, panic, worry, etc., but I knew I had to appear calm for the sake of my team and so that I could console the patient's daughter. While the paramedic spoke with the patient's daughter, I quickly made my way back to the infusion department to check on the nurses. This was the first death that the team experienced in our clinic. I could sense the shared purpose—nurses were in stages of shock and grief but were compassionately consoling the rest of the patients and continuing to diligently resume their nursing duties as best they could under the circumstances. Seeing the nurses carry on with their responsibilities while trying to process what just transpired gave me a surge of inner strength, since I realized I had to be strong for them to lean on me if needed.

"I mustered the focus to rise above the fear and sorrow I was feeling at the moment because I knew that's what each member of the care team was also doing, so that they could continue to provide the best care they could to their patients who were in the middle of their infusions. I returned to the lobby, where the patient's daughter was still speaking with the paramedics, and I stayed by her side to offer any support I could. A police officer also came on site in anticipation of the coroner arriving and he spoke with the patient's daughter briefly. Though I could not offer much other than my presence, I stayed with the daughter and spoke to her about her mother and listened as she expressed the range of feelings she was experiencing. At this early stage of the pandemic, social distancing was still strictly being enforced and I found it so difficult to keep from hugging her or reaching out to console her, as I normally would have done in such a situation pre-pandemic. In listening to the daughter, I learned that her mother had a premonition that she didn't have much time left despite going through chemotherapy and the early stage of her disease. Her mother had decided to change her advanced directive only a week prior and changed her status to DNR despite her family's protests. I must have talked with her for an hour and helped get her the resources she needed. She was adamant about driving home and did not want to break the news over the phone to her family at home. When she was composed enough to drive, she thanked me profusely and asked to send her gratitude to the nursing team for all that they did for her mother.

"Once I was able to return to the nursing team, I spent as much time as necessary with each of them so that they could express whatever they were feeling. We did a team debrief a few days later. When I reflect back on that day, I do not think I could have done what I did were it not for my staff. Their ability to carry on with compassionate nursing care with their patients despite just experiencing a traumatic event truly exemplified the spirit of nursing and bolstered me to be the leader they needed in the moment."

Gilanie D.
Manager, Med-Surg

Your Thoughts?

Pick one or more of these examples of peer wisdom about sisu to explore.

What lessons from your own experiences come to mind as you read these stories?

Q & Q: Quote and Question

Consider each quote about sisu and answer the follow-up question in light of your experiences.

> Q: "Most people never run far enough on their first wind to find out if they have a second wind."
>
> **William James**

Q: **Can you recall a time when "ran" so far in your practice that you experienced a second wind?**

....

....

....

....

> Q: "Let the globe, if nothing else say that this is true: that even as we grieved we grew. That even as we hurt we hoped. That even as we tired, we tried."
>
> **Amanda Gorman,** *The Hill We Climb*

Q: **Drawing from your own experiences as a leader, how would you interpret these words?**

....

....

....

....

> Q: "It may feel impossible but sometimes you have to take the first step—even before you are ready."
>
> **Sisu, the shape-shifting dragon,** *Raya and the Last Dragon*

Q: **Can you describe an experience when you faced your fears and moved toward meeting a challenge?**

....

....

Q: "In the depth of winter, I finally learned that within me there lay an invincible summer."

Albert Camus, *Journey to Tipasa*

Q: **Can you think of a time when you tapped into your invincible summer?**

Deep Dive Resources: Sisu

Books

Barnes, J. (2020). *Sisu: Find your resilience the Finnish way.* Sterling Ethos.

Dweck, C. S. (2006). *Mindset: The new psychology of success.* Ballantine Books.

Karjalainen, J. (2018). *Sisu: Resilience, belonging, purpose.* Chippenham.

Koppett, K. (2013). *Training to imagine: Practical improvisation techniques for trainers and managers.* Stylus Books.

Lahti, E. (2022). *Gentle power: A revolution in how we think, lead and succeed.* Soundstrue Incorporated.

Nyland, J. (2018). *Sisu: The Finnish art of courage.* Hachette Books.

Pantzar, K. T. (2018). *The Finnish way: Finding courage, wellness, and happiness through the power of sisu.* Tarcher Perigee.

Professional Journals, Chapters, and Scales

Cooperrider, D. L. (1990). Positive imagery, positive action: The affirmative basis of organizing. In S. Srivastva, & D. L. Cooperrider (Eds.), *Appreciative management and leadership: The power of positive thought and action in organizations* (pp. 91–125). Jossey Bass.

Cunha, M., Cunha, J., & Kamoche, K. (1999). Organizational improvisation: What, when, how, and why. *International Journal of Management, 1*(3), 299–341.

Fredrickson, B., & Joiner, T. (2002). Positive emotions trigger upward spirals toward emotional well-being. *Psychological Science, 13*(2), 172–175.

Gobbi, M. (2005). Nursing practice as bricoleur activity: A concept explored. *Nursing Inquiry, 12*(2), 117–125.

Lahti, E. (2019). Embodied fortitude: An introduction to the Finnish construct of sisu. *International Journal of Wellbeing*, *9*(1), 61–82.

Mackoff, B., & Triolo, P. (2008). Line of sight: The crucible in nurse manager engagement. *Nurse Leader*, *6*(4), 21–26.

Mathena, K. A. (2002). Nursing manager leadership skills. *Journal of Nursing Administration*, *32*(3), 136–142.

McCormick, M. (2001). Self-efficacy and leadership effectiveness: Applying social cognitive theory to leadership. *Journal of Leadership & Organizational Studies*, *8*(1), 22–33.

Rotter's *Locus of Control* scale. https://www.mccc.edu/~jenningh/Courses/documents/Rotter-locusofcontrolhandout.pdf

Videos and Audio

Mackoff, B. (n.d.). *Channeling inner strength through sisu* [Podcast]. American Organization of Nursing Leaders. https://www.aonl.org/resources/leading-through-crisis/strength-through-sisu

TEXxAlbany. (2011, February). *Kat Koppett: Improvisation: Not just for comedy anymore* [Video]. YouTube. https://www.youtube.com/watch?v=PZttwFLymJY

TEDxTurku. (2014, December). *Emilia Lahti: Sisu: Transforming barriers into frontiers* [Video]. YouTube. https://www.youtube.com/watch?v=UTIizGyf5kU

Ultrahabits. (2021, March). *Emilia Lahti: Turning pain into purpose* [Video]. YouTube. https://www.youtube.com/watch?v=iG2QvccDqfs

Figure Credit

Notes

Introduction

1. Mackoff, B. L., Glassman, K., & Budin, W. (2013). Developing a leadership laboratory for nurse managers based on lived experiences: A participatory action research model for leadership development. *The Journal of Nursing Administration*, *43*(9), 447–454.

2. Mackoff, B.L., & Triolo, P.K. (2008). Why do nurse managers stay? Building a model of engagement: Part 2, cultures of engagement. *The Journal of Nursing Administration*, *38*(4), 166–171.

3. Edmondson, C., McGough, K., Phillips, M., Blaine, Y., Scholl, D., & Mackoff, B. L. (2017). From a class to a community. A blueprint for a sustainable community of practice. *Nurse Leader, 15*(3), 179–183.

4. Mackoff, B.L., & Rasorg Weid, S. (2015, April). *Leder or leader? Empowering managers in Denmark.* Podium Presentation, AONE National Meeting, Phoenix, Arizona.

5. Lim, F.A., & Shi, T. (2013). Florence Nightingale: A pioneer of self-reflection. *Nursing, 43*(5), 1–3.

6. Bostridge, M. (2008). *Florence Nightingale: The making of an icon.* Farrar, Straus and Giroux.

7. Dewey, J. (1910). *How we think.* D.C. Heath.

8. Carper, B. A. (1978). Fundamental patterns of knowing in nursing. *Advances in Nursing Science, 1*(1), 13–23.

9. Schön, D. A. (1983). *The reflective practitioner.* Basic Books.

10. Benner, P. A. (1999). *From novice to expert: Excellence and power in clinical nursing practice.* Addison Wesley.

11. Schön, D. A., & Rein, M. (1994). *Frame reflection.* Basic Books.

12. Johns, C. (1995). The value of reflective practice for nursing. *Journal of Clinical Nursing, 4*(1), 23–30.

13. Gustafson, C., & Fagerberg, I. (2004). Reflection: The way to personal development? *Journal of Clinical Nursing, 13*(3), 271–280.

14. Atkins, S. (2004). Developing underlying skills in the move towards reflective practice. In C. Bulman & S. Schutz (Eds.), *Reflective practice in nursing* (3rd ed., pp. 23–52). Blackwell.

15. Atkins, S. (2008). Developing the skills for reflective practice. In S. Burns & C. Bulman (Eds.), *Reflective practice in nursing* (pp. 25–54). Blackwell Science.

16. Freshwater, D., Taylor, B. J., & Sherwood, G. D. (2009). *International textbook of reflective practice in nursing.* John Wiley.

17. Goulet, M. H., Larue, C., & Alderson, M. (2016). Reflective practice: A comparative dimensional analysis of the concept in nursing and education studies: A concept analysis of reflective practice. *Nursing Forum, 51*(2), 139–150.

18. Sherwood, R. G., & Horton-Deutsch, R. N. (2012). *Reflective practice: Transforming education and improving outcomes.* Sigma Tau International.

19 Patel, K., & Metersky, K. (2021). Reflective practice in nursing: A concept analysis. *International Journal of Nursing Knowledge*. Advance online publication. https://doi.org/10.1111/2047-3095.12350

20 Rieger, K. L., Chernomas, W. M., McMillan, D. E., & Morin, F. L. (2020). The arts as a catalyst for learning with undergraduate nursing students: Findings from a constructivist grounded theory study. *Arts & Health, 12*(3), 250–269.

21 Heckmann, B., Schols, J., & Halfens, R. A. (2015). A reflective framework to foster emotionally intelligent leadership in nursing. *Journal of Nursing Management, 23*(6), 744–753.

22 Horton-Deutsch, S., & Sherwood, G. (2008). Reflection: An educational strategy to develop emotionally competent nurse leaders. *Journal of Nursing Management, 16*(8), 946–949.

23 Vitello-Cicciu, J. (2002). Exploring emotional intelligence: Implications for nursing leaders. *The Journal of Nursing Administration, 32*(4), 203–210.

24 Coward, M. (2011). Does the use of reflective models restrict critical thinking and therefore learning in nurse education? What have we done? *Nurse Education Today, 31*(8), 883–886 (p. 884).

25 Schön, D. A. (1987). *Educating the reflective practitioner*, 28. Jossey Bass.

26 White, S., Fook, J., & Gardner, F. (2006). Critical reflection: A review of contemporary literature and understandings. In S. White, S. Fook & F. Gardner (Eds.), *Critical reflection in health and social care* (pp. 3–20). Maidenhead Open University Press.

27 Coward, M. (2011). Does the use of reflective models restrict critical thinking and therefore learning in nurse education? What have we done? *Nurse Education Today, 31*(8), 883–886 (p. 885).

28 Thompson, N., & Pascal, J. (2012). Developing critically reflective practice. *Reflective Practice: International and Multidisciplinary Perspectives, 13*(2), 311–325.

29 Reid, K., Flowers, P., & Larkin, M. (2005). Exploring lived experience. *Psychologist, 18*(1), 20–23.

30 Knowles, M. (1973). *The adult learner: A neglected species*. Gulf Publishing.

31 Graham-Hannah, D. J., Cathcart, E. B., Honan-Pellico, L., & Kunisch, J. (2017). Composing growth: Reflection through narrative. *Nursing Management, 48*(6), 40–45.

32 Cathcart, E., Greenspan, M., & Quin, M. (2010). The making of a nurse manager: The role of experiential learning in leadership development. *Journal of Nursing Management, 18*(4), 440–447.

33 Choperena, A., Oroviogoicoechea, C., Salcedo, A.Z., Moreno, I.O., & Jones, D. (2019). Nursing narratives and reflective practice: A theoretical review. *Journal of Advanced Nursing, 75*(8), 1637–1647.

34 Cathcart, E., & Greenspan, M. (2012). A new window into nurse manager development. *The Journal of Nursing Administration, 42*(12), 557–561.

Chapter 1

1 Loder, J. (1989). *The transformative moment*. Helmer and Howard.

2 Kegan, R. (1983). *The evolving self*. Harvard University Press.

3 Klein, G. (2013). *Seeing what others don't: The remarkable way we gain insights*. Perseus.

4 Underwood, P. (1994). *Three strands in the braid: A guide for enablers of learning*. Tribe of Two Press.

5   Bateson, G. (1991). *Further steps to an ecology of mind.* Harper Collins.

6   Robitallie, D. (2004). *Root cause analysis: Basic tools and techniques.* Paton Professional.

7   Thomas, R. (2008). *The crucibles of leadership: How to learn from experience to become a great leader.* Harvard Business School.

8   Stone, D., & Heen, S. (2014). *Thanks for the feedback: The science and art of receiving feedback well.* Viking.

9   Dweck, C. (2006). *Mindset: The new psychology of success.* Ballantine.

10   Whyte, D. (2001). *Crossing the unknown sea: Work as a pilgrimage of identity.* Riverhead Books.

Chapter 2

1   Maslow, A. H. (2013). *A theory of human motivation.* Martino Publishing.

2   Skinner, B. F. (1976). *About behaviorism.* Vintage Books.

3   Mackoff, B., & Triolo, P. (2008). Line of sight: The crucible in nurse manager engagement. *Nurse Leader, 6*(4), 21–26.

4   Mackoff, B. (2011). *Nurse manager engagement: Strategies for excellence and commitment,* 171. Jones & Bartlett.

5   Sinek, S. (2009). S*tart with why.* Penguin.

6   Mackoff, B. (2011). *Nurse manager engagement: Strategies for excellence and commitment,* 11, 17. Jones & Bartlett.

7   Whyte, D. (2001). *Crossing the unknown sea: Work as a pilgrimage of identity.* Riverhead Books.

8   Eileen Magri, PhD, in private conversation, October 2012.

9   Kegan, R., Lahey, L. L. (2001). *How the way we talk can change the way we work: Seven languages for transformation,* 92. Wiley.

10   Mackoff, B., & Wenet, G. (2004). *The inner work of leaders: Leadership as a habit of mind.* Amacom.

11   Chapman, G., & White, P. (2019). *The 5 languages of appreciation in the workplace: Empowering organizations by encouraging people.* Northfield Publishing.

12   Schein, E. (2013). *Humble inquiry.* Berrett-Koehler.

13   Pink, D. (2009). *Drive: The surprising truth about what motivates us.* Riverhead Books.

14   Erickson, E. (1950). *Childhood and society.* Norton.

15   McAdams, D. A., & de St Aubin, E. (1998). The anatomy of generativity. In D. A. McAdams & E. de St Aubin (Eds.), *Generativity and adult development.* APA Press.

16   Weiner, B. (1985). An attributional theory of achievement motivation and emotion. *Psychological Review, 92*(4), 548–573.

17   Cooperrider, D., & Srivastva, S. *Appreciative management and leadership: The power of positive thought and action in organizations.* Jossey Bass.

Chapter 3

1   Mackoff, B., & Triolo, P. (2008). Why do nurses stay? Building a model of engagement. *Journal of Nursing Administration*, *38*(3), 118–124.

2   Chreim, S., & Langley, A. (2013). Leadership boundary work in therapeutic teams. *Leadership*, *9*(2), 201–228.

3   Tawwab, N. (2021). *Set boundaries, find peace*. Penguin.

4   Adams, J. *Boundary issues: Using boundary intelligence*. Wiley and Sons.

5   Black, J., & Enns, G. (1997). *Better boundaries: Owning and treasuring your life*. Raincoast Books.

6   Mackoff, B. (2011). *Nurse manager engagement: Strategies for excellence and commitment*. Jones & Bartlett.

7   Hartmann, E. (1991). *Boundaries in the mind: A new psychology of personality*. Basic Books.

8   Bowen, M. (1985). On the differentiation of self. In M. Bowen (Ed.), *Family therapy in clinical practice* (p. 478). Rowman & Littlefield Publishers, Inc.

9   Ormond, L. (1994). Developing emotional insulation. *International Journal of Group Psychotherapy*, *44*(3), 361–375.

10 Covey, S. (2020). *The 7 habits of highly effective people*. Simon & Shuster.

11 Heifetz, R., & Linksy, M. (2002). *Leadership on the line*. Harvard Business School.

12 Buchanan, G., & Seligman, M. (2009). *Explanatory style*. Routledge.

13 Angelou, M. (2019). *Maya Angelou wisdom* (Pocket Edition). Hardie Grant.

Chapter 4

1   Kipling, R. (1989). *Rudyard Kipling: Complete verses*. Anchor Books.

2   Salovey, P., & Mayer, J. D. (1990). Emotional intelligence. *Imagination, Cognition and Personality*, *9*(3), 185–211.

3   Goleman, D. (2001). *Working with emotional intelligence*. Bantam Books.

4   Muraven, M. R., & Baumeister, R. F. (2000). Self-regulation and depletion of limited resources: Does self-control resemble a muscle? *Psychological Bulletin*, *126*(2), 247–259.

5   Hoyle, R. (2010). Personality and self-regulation. In R. Hoyle (Ed.), *Handbook of personality and self-regulation* (pp. 1–18). Blackwell Publishing.

6   Patterson, K., Grenny, J., McMillan, R., & Switzler, A. (2012). *Crucial conversations: Tools for talking when the stakes are high*. McGraw Hill.

7   Private conversation with Kristiina Junttila, PhD, director of Nursing Research Centre, Helsinki University Hospital, Helsinki, Finland, May 2017.

8   James, W. (1950). *The principles of psychology*. Holt.

9   Bieleke, M., Lucas, K., & Gollwitzer, P. (2021). If-then planning. *European Review of Social Psychology*, *32*(1), 88–122.

10 Beck, A. T. (1976). *Cognitive therapies and emotional disorders*. New American Library.

11 Burns, D. D. (1980). *Feeling good: The new mood therapy*. New American Library.

12 Mackoff, B., & Wenet, G. (2004). *The inner work of leaders*, 129. Amacom.

13 Lynn, A. (2002). *The emotional intelligence activity book.* HRD Press.

14 Glaser, J. (2014). *Conversational intelligence.* Bibliomotion.

15 Kegan, R. (1983). *The evolving self.* Harvard University Press.

16 Seligman, M. E. P., & Elder, G. H. (1986). Explanatory style across life span: Achievement and health. In A. Sorenson, F. E. Weinert, & L. Sherrod (Eds.), *Learned helplessness and life span development* (pp. 377–427). Erlbaum.

17 Stosny, S. (2004). *The powerful self.* BookSurge.

18 Mackoff, B. (2011). *Nurse manager engagement: Strategies for excellence and commitment.* Jones & Bartlett.

Chapter 5

1 Erickson, E. (1963). *Childhood and society.* Norton.

2 de St. Aubin, E., & McAdams, D. P. (1995). The relations of generative concern and generative action to personality traits, satisfaction/happiness with life, and ego development. *Journal of Adult Development, 2*, 99–112.

3 Kotre, J. (1988). *Outliving the self: Generativity and the interpretation of lives.* Johns Hopkins University Press.

4 McAdams, D. P., & Logan, R. L. (2004). What is generativity? In E. de St. Aubin, D. P. McAdams, & T.-C. Kim (Eds.), *The generative society: Caring for future generations* (pp. 15–31). American Psychological Association.

5 McAdams, D. P., & de St. Aubin, E. (1998). *Generativity and adult development: How and why we care for the next generation.* The American Psychological Association.

6 Grossman, S. (2013). *Mentoring in nursing.* Springer.

7 Vance, C. (2005). Leader as mentor. In H. R. Feldman & M. J. Greenberg (Eds.), *Educating nurses for leadership* (pp. 80–97). Springer Publishing Company.

8 McAdams, D. P., & de St. Aubin, E. (1992). A theory of generativity and its assessment through self-report, behavioral acts, and narrative themes in autobiography. *Journal of Personality and Social Psychology, 62*(6), 1003–1015.

9 McCloughen, A., O'Brien, L., & Jackson, D. (2011). Nurse leader mentor as a mode of being: Findings from an Australian hermeneutic phenomenological study. *Journal of Nursing Scholarship, 43*(1), 97–104.

10 Mackoff, B. (2011). *Nurse manager engagement: Strategies for excellence and commitment.* Jones and Bartlett.

11 Thoreau, H. D. (1854). *Walden: Or life in the woods.* Ticknor and Fields.

12 Kotre, J. (1999). *Make it count: How to generate a legacy that gives meaning to your life.* Free Press.

13 Kotre, J. (1999). *Make it count: How to generate a legacy that gives meaning to your life.* Free Press.

14 Nightingale, F. (1969). *Notes on nursing.* Dover Publications.

15 Ready, D. (2002). How storytelling builds next-generation leaders. *MIT Sloan Management Review, 43*(4), 63–69.

16   Mackoff, B. (2011). *Nurse manager engagement: Strategies for excellence and commitment.* Jones and Bartlett, p. 68.

17   Jackson, D. (2008). Random acts of guidance: Personal reflections on professional generosity. *Journal of Clinical Nursing, 17*(20), 2669–2670.

18   Huber, D. (2004). *Leadership and nursing care management.* Elsevier.

19   King, T. (2000). Paradigms of Canadian nurse managers: Lenses for viewing leadership and management. *Canadian Journal of Nursing Leadership, 13*(1), 15–20.

20   Dweck, C. (2006). *Mindset: The new psychology of success.* Ballantine.

Chapter 6

1   Stefancyk, A., Hancock, B., & Meadows, M. (2012). The nurse manager: Change agent, change coach or both? *Nursing Admin Quarterly, 36*(1), 1–5.

2   Goleman, D. (2000). *Working with emotional intelligence.* Bantam.

3   Heifetz, R. A., Linsky, M., & Grashow, A. (2009). *The practice of adaptive leadership: Tools and tactics for changing your organization and the world.* Harvard Business Press.

4   Heifetz, R. A., Linsky, M., & Grashow, A. (2009). *The practice of adaptive leadership: Tools and tactics for changing your organization and the world.* Harvard Business Press.

5   Bowie, D. (1971). Changes [Song]. On *Hunky Dory.* RCA Records.

6   Fugate, M., & Kinicki, A. (2017). *Organizational behavior: A practical, problem-solving approach.* McGraw Hill.

7   Lencioni, N. (2000). *The five dysfunctions of a team.* Jossey Bass.

8   Edmondson, A. (2018). *The fearless organization: Creating psychological safety in the workplace for learning, innovation, and growth.* John Wiley & Sons.

9   Holbeche, L. (2006). *Understanding change: Theory, implementation and success.* Elsevier.

10 Balfour, M., & Clarke, C. (2001). Searching for sustainable change. *Journal of Clinical Nursing, 10*(1), 44–50.

11 Eliot, T. S. (1974). *The four quartets collected poems 1909–1962.* Faber & Faber Ltd.

12 Lawrence-Lightfoot, S. (2012). *Exit: The endings that set us free.* Farrar, Straus and Giroux.

13 Sinek, S. (2011). *Start with why: How great leaders inspire everyone to take action.* Penguin Books.

14 Kotter, J., & Cohen, D. (2012). *The heart of change.* Harvard Business Review.

15 Kegan, R., & Laskow-Lahey, L. (2009). *Immunity to change.* Harvard Business Press.

16 Ryan, R., & Deci, E. (2017). *Basic psychological needs in motivation, development and wellness.* Guilford Press.

17 Deming, W. E. (1991). *Out of the crisis, 1986.* Massachusetts Institute of Technology Center for Advanced Engineering Study (pp. 13, 507).

18 Dyer, J., Gregerson, H., & Christensen, C. (2011). *The Innovator's DNA.* Harvard Business Review Press.

19 Musselwhite, C., & Jones, R. (2004). *Dangerous opportunity: Making change work.* XLibris.

20 Lueger, G. (2006). Solution-focused management: Towards a theory of positive difference. In G. Lueger & H.-P. Korn (Eds.), *Solution-focused management* (pp. 1–13). Rainer Hampp Verlag.

21 Cooperrider, D., Whitney, D., & Stavros, J. (2008). *Appreciative inquiry handbook for leaders of change.* Berrett Koehler.

22 de Shazer, S., Berg, I. K., Lipchik, E., Nunnally, E., Molnar, A., & Gingerich, W. (1986). Brief therapy: Focused solution-development. *Family Process, 25*(2), 207–222.

23 Bateson, G. (1972). *Steps to an ecology of mind: Collected essays in anthropology, psychiatry, evolution, and epistemology.* University of Chicago Press.

24 Duclos, M. (2006). Solution focused leadership through appreciation. In G. Lueger & H.-P. Korn (Eds.), *Solution-focused management* (pp. 123–134). Rainer Hampp Verlag.

25 McKergow, M., & Clarke, J. (2007). *Solutions focus working: 80 real life lessons for successful organizational change.* Solutions Books.

26 Kegan, R., & Laskow-Lahey, L. (2001). *How the way we talk can change the way we work.* Jossey-Bass.

27 Cooperrider, D., & Srivastva, S. (1987). Appreciative inquiry in organizational life. In R. Woodman & W. Pasmore (Eds.), *Research in organizational change and development* (pp. 129–169). JAI Press.

28 Marchionni, C., & Richer, M. C. (2007). Using appreciative inquiry to promote evidence-based practice in nursing: The glass is more than half full. *Nursing Leadership, 20*(3), 86–97.

29 May, N., & Becker, D. (2011). *Appreciative inquiry in healthcare.* Crown Custom.

Chapter 7

1 Lahti, E. (2019). Embodied fortitude: An introduction to the Finnish construct of sisu. *International Journal of Wellbeing, 9*(1), 61–82.

2 Mackoff, B. (2020). Channeling inner strength through sisu [Podcast]. American Organization of Nursing Leaders.

3 Strode, H. (1940, January 14). Sisu: A word that explains Finland. *The New York Times,* 4–5.

4 TEDxTurku. (2014, December). *Emilia Lahti: Sisu: Transforming barriers into frontiers* [Video]. YouTube. https://www.youtube.com/watch?v=UTIizGyf5kU

5 Amato-Henderson, S., Slade, D., & Kemppainen, A. (2014). Measuring sisu: Development of a tool to measure mental toughness in academia. *Proceedings of the Human Factors and Ergonomics Society Annual Meeting, 58*(1), 1434–1436.

6 Henttonen, P., Määttänen, I., & Hofericher, F. (2021, July 7). Internal and external validation of the Sisu Scale in a German sample [Paper presentation]. International Conference of the Stress Trauma Anxiety and Resilience Society, Haifa, Israel.

7 Henttonen, P., Määttänen, I., Makkonen, E., Honka, A., Seppälä, V., Närväinen, J., & Lahti, E. E. (2022). A measure for assessment of beneficial and harmful fortitude: Development and initial validation of the Sisu Scale. *PsyArXiv.* Advance online publication. https://doi.org/10.31234/osf.io/7nptw

8   Private conversation with Emilia Elisabet Lahti, April 20, 2020.

9   Mackoff, B., & Wenet, G. (2004). *The inner work of leaders: Leadership as a habit of mind*, 179. Amacom.

10   Gelb, M. (1998). *How to think like Leonardo da Vinci*, 58. Delacorte Press.

11   Benefiel, M. (2008). Using discernment to make better business decisions. In G. Flynn (Ed.), *Leadership and Business Ethics* (pp. 31–38). Springer Netherlands.

12   Weick, K., Sutcliffe, M., & Obstfeld, D. (2005). Organizing and the process of sensemaking. *Organization Science, 16*(4), 409–421.

13   Collins, J. (2001). *Good to great.* Harper Collins.

14   Traüffer Hazel, C. V., Bekker, C., & Bocârnea, M. (2010). A three-factor measure of discernment. *Leadership & Organization Development Journal, 31*(3), 263–284.

15   Miller, K. (2020). Discernment in management and organizations *Journal of Management, Spirituality & Religion, 17*(5), 373–402.

16   Camus, A. (1955). *The myth of Sisyphus and other essays.* Knopf.

17   Camus, A. (1955). *The myth of Sisyphus and other essays.* Knopf.

18   McCormick, M. (2001). Self-efficacy and leadership effectiveness: Applying social cognitive theory to leadership. *Journal of Leadership & Organizational Studies, 8*(1), 22–33.

19   Popper, M., & Mayseless, O. (2007). The building blocks of leader development: A psychological conceptual framework. *Leadership & Organization Development Journal, 28*(7), 664–684.

20   Mathena, K. (2002). Nursing manager leadership skills. *Journal of Nursing Administration, 32*(3), 136–142.

21   Bandura, A. (1995). *Self-efficacy in changing societies.* Cambridge University Press.

22   Rotter, J. B. (1966). Generalized expectancies for internal versus external control of reinforcement. *Psychological Monographs, 80*(1), 1–28.

23   Maxwell, J. (2007). *Failing forward.* Thomas Nelson.

24   Dweck, C. S. (2006). *Mindset: The new psychology of success.* Random House.

25   Stewart, G., Courtright, S., & Manz, C. (2011). Self-leadership: A multilevel review. *Journal of Management 37*(1), 185–222.

26   Manz, C., & Neck, C. P. (1991). Inner leadership: Creating productive thought patterns. *Academy of Management Executives, 5*(3), 87–95.

27   Neck, C.P., & Manz, C. (1992). Thought self-leadership: The influence of self-talk and mental imagery on performance. *Journal of Organizational Behavior, 13*(7), 681–699.

28   Rogelberg, S., Justice, L., Braddy, P. W., Paustian-Underdahl, S. C., Heggestad, E., Shanock, L., Baran, B. E., Beck, T., Long, S., Andrew, A., Altman, D. G., Fleenor, J. W. (2013). The executive mind: Leader self-talk, effectiveness, and strain. *Journal of Managerial Psychology, 28*(2), 183–201.

29   Houghto, J., & Neck, C. (2002). The Revised Self-Leadership Questionnaire: Testing a hierarchical factor structure for self-leadership. *Journal of Managerial Psychology, 17*(8), 672–691.

30   Mackoff, B., & Triolo, P. (2008). Line of sight: The crucible in nurse manager engagement. *Nurse Leader, 6*(4), 21–26.

31   Bennis, W. (1994). *An invented life; reflections on leadership and change.* Basic Books.

32   Weick, K. (1979). *The social psychology of organizing.* Addison Wesley.

33 Lahti, E. (2013, December 2).The brilliance of the dream: Introducing sisu as an action mindset. *The Creativity Post.*

34 Cooperrider, D. (1990). Positive imagery, positive action: The affirmative basis of organizing. In S. Srivastva, D. L. Cooperrider (Eds.), *Appreciative management and leadership: The power of positive thought and action in organizations* (pp. 91–125). Jossey Bass.

35 Levi-Strauss, C. (1968). *The savage mind.* University of Chicago Press.

36 Baker, T., & Nelson, R. (2005). Creating something from nothing: Resource construction through entrepreneurial bricolage. *Administrative Science Quarterly, 50*(3), 329–366.

37 Gobbi, M. (2005). Nursing practice as bricoleur activity: A concept explored. *Nursing Inquiry, 12*(2), 117–125.

38 Mackoff, B. (2011). *Nurse manager engagement: Strategies for excellence and commitment.* Jones and Bartlett.

39 Koppett, K. (2013). Training to imagine: Practical improvisation techniques for trainers and managers. Stylus Books.

40 Spolin, V. (1983). *Improvisation for theater.* Northwestern University.

41 Levi-Strauss, C. (1968). *The savage mind*, 17. University of Chicago Press.

Index

About the Author

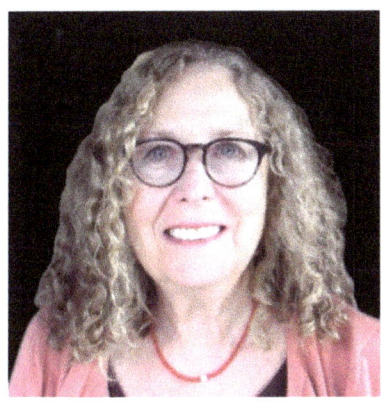

Dr. Barbara Mackoff is a consulting psychologist, author, leadership educator and keynote speaker. She is a Fulbright specialist and a senior faculty member at The American Organization of Nursing Leaders. She develops and facilitates AONL'S national online Leadership Laboratory for Nurse Managers.

She has designed and facilitated leadership development programs for nurse leaders worldwide, including Gentofte Hospital in Copenhagen, Helsinki University Hospital in Finland, and Zurich University Hospital in Switzerland.

Dr. Mackoff was principal investigator of a national research study of nurse manager engagement funded by the Robert Wood Johnson Foundation.

She is the author of six books, including *Nurse Manager Engagement, The Inner Work of Leaders,* and *The Art of Self-Renewal.* Her research has been published in *The Journal of Nursing Administration* and *Nurse Leader.* Her work has been featured in *The New York Times, USA Today,* and *The Washington Post,* and she has appeared on *The Today Show, CBS Morning News,* and NPR's *All Things Considered.*

Educated at Harvard University, Dr. Mackoff has held educational and clinical appointments at the University of Washington Department of Psychiatry and Behavioral Sciences and the Schools of Nursing at Adelphi University and Molloy College in New York.

She can be contacted at blmackoff@gmail.com.